SOMATIC EXERCISES
FOR BEGINNERS

Achieve Mind-Body Balance, Lose Weight, and
Relieve Chronic Pain, Tension and Stress
in Just 10 Minutes a Day

Lara Namaskar

TABLE OF CONTENTS

INTRODUCTION TO "SOMATIC EXERCISES FOR BEGINNERS"

What Are Somatic Exercises?

As we embark on the journey of exploring somatic exercises, it's essential to grasp the essence of this transformative practice. Somatic exercises, rooted in the profound connection between the mind and body, offer a gateway to self-discovery and holistic well-being. Let's delve into the intricate tapestry of somatic movement, where each stretch, each breath, becomes a dance of liberation and awareness.

At its core, somatic exercises embody the philosophy that our bodies are not mere vessels to be manipulated but sacred landscapes to be revered and understood. Unlike conventional workouts that focus solely on external outcomes, somatic exercises invite us to journey inward, to listen intently to the whispers of our muscles, bones, and breath.

Imagine yourself standing at the threshold of your inner sanctuary, where movement becomes a language of introspection and healing. Somatic exercises encompass a diverse range of practices, from gentle stretches to dynamic sequences, all designed to awaken dormant layers of sensation and vitality within.

One of the defining characteristics of somatic exercises is their emphasis on embodiment—the art of fully inhabiting our physical form. Through mindful movement and conscious breathing, we cultivate a deep sense of presence, anchoring ourselves in the present moment. Each stretch becomes an invitation to be here now, to release the burdens of the past and the anxieties of the future.

Moreover, somatic exercises offer a unique opportunity to unravel the patterns of tension and resistance that accumulate in our bodies over time. In today's fast-paced world, where stress and sedentary lifestyles reign supreme, our muscles often bear the brunt of our unprocessed emotions and unmet needs. Somatic exercises serve as a gentle antidote to this modern affliction, allowing us to unravel the knots of chronic tension and reclaim our innate capacity for ease and grace.

As we engage in somatic exercises, we become alchemists of sensation, transmuting discomfort into liberation and stiffness into suppleness. Each movement becomes a sacred ritual, a celebration of the body's inherent wisdom and resilience. We learn to move not out of obligation or force but out of love and reverence for this miraculous vessel that carries us through life's journey.

Furthermore, somatic exercises provide a profound gateway to self-awareness and self-expression. As we attune ourselves to the subtleties of sensation, we develop a nuanced understanding of our bodies' unique needs and desires. We learn to move with intention and integrity, honoring the wisdom encoded in every cell and sinew.

In essence, somatic exercises offer a holistic path to health and vitality—one that integrates the physical, emotional, and spiritual dimensions of our being. Through mindful movement and embodied awareness, we reclaim our birthright as sovereign beings, capable of experiencing profound joy and aliveness in every moment.

Somatic exercises invite us to embark on a sacred journey of self-discovery and transformation—a journey where movement becomes medicine, and the body becomes a temple of awakening. Let us embrace this profound practice with open hearts and open minds, knowing that within the depths of our own being lies the key to wholeness and well-being.

Benefits of Somatic Movement for Beginners

Exploring the world of somatic movement opens a gateway to a realm of profound benefits, especially for those new to this transformative prac-

tice. As we embark on this journey of self-discovery and embodied awareness, let us unravel the myriad ways in which somatic movement can en-
rich our lives and enhance our well-being.

At its core, somatic movement offers a holistic approach to health and
vitality—one that transcends the limitations of conventional exercise reg-
imens. Unlike traditional workouts that focus solely on external outcomes such as muscle strength or cardiovascular fitness, somatic movement addresses the root causes of tension and imbalance within the
body.

One of the most profound benefits of somatic movement for beginners
is its ability to increase body awareness and mindfulness. Through gentle,
exploratory movements and focused attention, we cultivate a deep
sense of presence and connection with our bodies. We learn to listen to
the subtle whispers of sensation, tuning into the wisdom encoded in
every muscle fiber and joint.

Moreover, somatic movement serves as a powerful tool for stress reduction and relaxation. In today's fast-paced world, where chronic stress has
become a ubiquitous companion, somatic exercises offer a sanctuary of
peace and tranquility. By engaging in slow, mindful movements and conscious breathing practices, we activate the body's relaxation response,
calming the nervous system and soothing frayed nerves.

Furthermore, somatic movement promotes greater flexibility and mobility, helping beginners to unlock the full potential of their bodies. Through
gentle stretching and dynamic movement sequences, we release tight
muscles and lubricate stiff joints, allowing for greater freedom of movement and ease in daily activities.

Additionally, somatic movement can be a potent ally in the journey towards emotional healing and self-discovery. As we delve into the depths
of our own embodied experience, we may uncover long-held emotional
patterns and traumas stored within the body. Through somatic practices
such as emotional release techniques and guided movement explorations, we create a safe container for processing and integrating these bur-
ied emotions, paving the way for greater emotional resilience and well-
being.

Moreover, somatic movement offers a pathway to improved posture and body alignment—an often overlooked aspect of overall health and well-being. Through targeted exercises that address imbalances and asymmetries in the body, beginners can gradually realign their posture, reducing strain and tension in the muscles and joints.

Furthermore, somatic movement fosters a deep sense of empowerment and agency within beginners, allowing them to reclaim ownership of their bodies and their health. By cultivating a mindful and compassionate relationship with their bodies, beginners learn to trust in the innate wisdom of their own embodied experience, paving the way for greater self-confidence and self-esteem.

The benefits of somatic movement for beginners are vast and multifaceted, encompassing physical, emotional, and spiritual dimensions of well-being. Through mindful movement, conscious breathing, and embodied awareness, beginners can unlock the full potential of their bodies and cultivate a profound sense of vitality and aliveness in every moment. Let us embrace this transformative practice with open hearts and open minds, knowing that within the depths of our own embodied experience lies the key to radiant health and well-being.

Understanding Your Body's Wisdom: A Beginner's Perspective

Delving into the realm of somatic movement, one cannot help but be captivated by the profound wisdom that resides within the body. As beginners embark on this journey of self-discovery and embodied awareness, they are invited to explore the depths of their own being with a sense of curiosity and wonder.

From the moment we take our first breath, our bodies become vessels of wisdom, each cell pulsating with the rhythm of life itself. Yet, in the hustle and bustle of modern existence, we often find ourselves disconnected from this innate source of guidance and insight. Somatic movement offers a pathway back to our roots, a journey of rediscovery that begins with a simple yet profound shift in perspective.

For beginners, understanding the body's wisdom is akin to embarking on a voyage of self-exploration—a journey into the depths of one's own being. It is an invitation to peel back the layers of conditioning and societal norms that have shaped our perception of ourselves and our bodies, and to reconnect with the primal intelligence that lies at the core of our being. At the heart of somatic movement lies the principle of embodied awareness—a state of being in which we are fully present and attuned to the sensations and signals of our own bodies. As beginners cultivate this awareness, they begin to develop a deeper understanding of the intricate language of the body—a language that speaks in whispers of sensation, movement, and breath.

Moreover, understanding the body's wisdom is about learning to trust in the innate intelligence of the body—to recognize that it holds the answers to our deepest questions and concerns. As beginners engage in somatic practices such as gentle movement explorations and mindful breathing exercises, they learn to listen to the subtle cues and signals that arise from within, trusting in the body's innate ability to heal and regenerate itself.

Furthermore, understanding the body's wisdom is about honoring the interconnectedness of mind, body, and spirit—a recognition that we are not separate beings, but rather integral parts of a greater whole. As beginners cultivate this awareness, they begin to appreciate the profound interconnectedness of all aspects of their being, and to recognize that true healing and transformation can only occur when we address the body as a whole.

In essence, understanding your body's wisdom is about embracing a paradigm shift—a shift from seeing the body as a mere machine to be controlled and manipulated, to recognizing it as a sacred vessel of wisdom and intelligence. It is an invitation to journey inward, to explore the vast depths of our own being with a sense of reverence and awe.

As beginners embark on this journey of self-discovery and embodied awareness, they are reminded that they are not alone—that they are part of a larger tapestry of life, woven together by the threads of shared humanity. And as they navigate the twists and turns of this sacred journey, they are guided by the timeless wisdom that resides within their own bodies—a wisdom that has been waiting patiently to be rediscovered and embraced.

Overcoming Common Challenges in Starting a Somatic Practice

Embarking on a journey of somatic practice is akin to setting sail on a voyage of self-discovery and transformation. Yet, like any journey worth undertaking, it is not without its challenges. As beginners take their first steps into the realm of somatic movement, they may encounter a myriad of obstacles along the way. However, with patience, perseverance, and a willingness to embrace the process, these challenges can be transformed into opportunities for growth and learning.

One of the most common challenges that beginners face when starting a somatic practice is the tendency to approach it with a goal-oriented mindset. In our fast-paced, results-driven culture, we are conditioned to seek instant gratification and tangible outcomes. However, somatic movement is not about achieving a specific end goal, but rather about cultivating a deeper awareness and connection with the body. As beginners learn to let go of the need to "succeed" or "achieve," they can begin to embrace the process of exploration and discovery, allowing themselves to be fully present in each moment.

Another common challenge for beginners is the discomfort that arises when confronting long-held patterns of tension and resistance within the body. Somatic movement invites us to explore the depths of our own being, to peel back the layers of conditioning and societal norms that have shaped our perception of ourselves and our bodies. Yet, this process of exploration can be unsettling, as we come face to face with the physical and emotional baggage that we have been carrying for so long. However, by approaching this discomfort with compassion and curiosity, beginners can begin to unravel the knots of tension that bind them, allowing for greater freedom and ease of movement.

Furthermore, beginners may struggle with the concept of "letting go" and surrendering to the innate intelligence of the body. In a culture that values control and mastery, the idea of relinquishing control can be daunting. However, somatic movement teaches us that true healing and transformation occur when we learn to trust in the wisdom of the body— to listen to its cues and signals, and to follow its lead with openness and receptivity. By cultivating a sense of trust and surrender, beginners can tap into the inherent healing power that resides within their own bodies, allowing for profound shifts to occur on physical, emotional, and spiritual levels.

Additionally, beginners may encounter challenges related to consistency and commitment in their somatic practice. In our busy and hectic lives, finding the time and energy to dedicate to regular practice can be challenging. However, establishing a consistent routine is essential for deepening one's somatic experience and reaping the full benefits of the practice. By setting realistic goals and creating a supportive environment for practice, beginners can overcome this challenge and cultivate a sustainable somatic practice that enriches their lives on a daily basis.

While starting a somatic practice may pose its fair share of challenges, it is important for beginners to approach these obstacles with patience, perseverance, and an open heart. By embracing the process of exploration and discovery, cultivating trust in the wisdom of the body, and establishing a consistent practice routine, beginners can overcome these challenges and unlock the transformative power of somatic movement in their lives.

Setting Intentions and Goals for Your Somatic Journey

Embarking on a somatic journey is akin to setting sail on an odyssey of self-discovery and transformation. As we step onto the path of somatic movement, we are invited to embark on a profound exploration of the body, mind, and spirit—a journey that holds the promise of healing, growth, and awakening. Yet, like any journey worth undertaking, it is essential to set intentions and goals that will guide us along the way, helping to illuminate our path and keep us focused on our destination.

Setting intentions for our somatic practice is like planting seeds in the fertile soil of our consciousness—seeds that will germinate and blossom into the fruits of our labor. These intentions act as beacons of light, illuminating our path and guiding us toward our desired destination. Whether our intention is to cultivate greater flexibility, alleviate chronic pain, or simply deepen our connection with ourselves, setting clear and concise intentions allows us to harness the power of our subconscious mind and align our actions with our deepest desires.

When setting intentions for our somatic journey, it is important to approach the process with clarity, mindfulness, and authenticity. Rather than setting goals based on external expectations or societal norms, we must take the time to tune into our innermost desires and aspirations, listening deeply to the whispers of our soul. What is it that we truly long for? What do we hope to gain from our somatic practice? By taking the time to reflect on these questions and articulate our intentions with sincerity and conviction, we can set the stage for profound transformation and growth.

In addition to setting intentions, it is also important to establish clear and actionable goals that will serve as milestones on our somatic journey. While intentions provide us with a sense of direction and purpose, goals offer us tangible markers of progress and achievement, helping to keep us motivated and focused on our path. Whether our goals are to master a specific somatic technique, overcome a particular challenge, or simply cultivate a greater sense of well-being, it is essential to make them specific, measurable, achievable, relevant, and time-bound (SMART).

As we embark on our somatic journey, it is natural to encounter obstacles and challenges along the way. However, by setting clear intentions and goals, we can navigate these challenges with grace and resilience, using them as opportunities for growth and learning. When faced with setbacks or roadblocks, we can refer back to our intentions and goals, drawing strength and inspiration from the vision of our desired outcome. In this way, setting intentions and goals acts as a powerful tool for staying aligned with our purpose and staying committed to our somatic practice, even in the face of adversity.

Moreover, setting intentions and goals for our somatic journey is not a one-time event but an ongoing process of reflection, refinement, and evolution. As we progress on our path, our intentions and goals may shift and evolve, reflecting our changing needs, desires, and aspirations. It is important to revisit our intentions and goals regularly, reassessing our priorities and adjusting our course as needed. In doing so, we can ensure that our somatic practice remains dynamic, vibrant, and aligned with our deepest values and aspirations.

By clarifying our intentions, articulating our goals, and staying aligned with our purpose, we can navigate the challenges of our journey with grace and resilience, ultimately realizing our full potential and experiencing profound healing and transformation on all levels of our being.

THE FOUNDATIONS OF SOMATIC MOVEMENT

1.1 Exploring the Mind-Body Connection

Embarking on a journey of exploring the mind-body connection is akin to delving into the depths of our own consciousness—a journey of profound self-discovery and transformation. At the heart of somatic movement lies the understanding that the mind and body are not separate entities but rather interconnected aspects of our being, each influencing and shaping the other in profound ways. As we embark on this journey of exploration, we are invited to deepen our understanding of this intricate relationship, unlocking the secrets of our own inner landscape and tapping into the vast potential of our embodied experience.

Central to exploring the mind-body connection is the recognition that our bodies are not simply mechanical vessels but dynamic expressions of our thoughts, emotions, and beliefs. Every sensation, every movement, every gesture carries with it a wealth of meaning and significance, reflecting the complex interplay between our inner world and outer reality. By cultivating greater awareness of these subtle nuances and learning to listen to the wisdom of our bodies, we can uncover deep insights into our own psyche and gain a deeper understanding of ourselves.

One of the most powerful tools for exploring the mind-body connection is the practice of mindfulness—a state of open-hearted awareness and non-judgmental presence. Through mindfulness, we can cultivate a deep sense of attunement to the present moment, allowing us to fully experience and embrace the richness of our embodied experience. By bringing mindful awareness to our thoughts, sensations, and emotions, we can begin to unravel the intricate tapestry of our inner landscape, gaining insight into the hidden patterns and conditioning that shape our behavior and perceptions.

In addition to mindfulness, somatic movement offers a rich array of practices and techniques for exploring the mind-body connection. From gentle movement explorations to dynamic somatic exercises, these practices provide us with a powerful means of accessing the wisdom of our bodies and uncovering the deeper layers of our own being. Through somatic movement, we can learn to inhabit our bodies more fully, awakening to the subtle sensations and nuances that lie beneath the surface of our awareness.

One of the key principles underlying the mind-body connection is the concept of embodied cognition—the idea that our thoughts and perceptions are intimately linked to our bodily experience. According to embodied cognition theory, our bodies serve as a gateway to our minds, shaping our thoughts, emotions, and perceptions in profound and often unconscious ways. By exploring the mind-body connection, we can begin to unravel these hidden connections, gaining insight into the ways in which our physical experiences shape our mental and emotional states.

Moreover, exploring the mind-body connection offers profound implications for our health and well-being. Research has shown that cultivating a strong mind-body connection can have a wide range of benefits, including reduced stress, improved mood, enhanced cognitive function, and increased resilience to illness and disease. By learning to listen to the wisdom of our bodies and aligning our actions with our innermost needs and desires, we can unlock the healing power that lies within us and cultivate a greater sense of vitality and well-being.

Exploring the mind-body connection is a journey of profound self-discovery and transformation—one that offers us the opportunity to deepen our understanding of ourselves and unlock the hidden potential of our embodied experience. Through practices such as mindfulness and somatic movement, we can learn to listen to the wisdom of our bodies, unraveling the mysteries of our own inner landscape and tapping into the boundless potential that lies within us. As we embark on this journey, may we approach it with curiosity, openness, and reverence, honoring the sacred union of mind and body and embracing the limitless possibilities that lie ahead.

1.2 Principles of Somatic Education: A Beginner's Guide

Rooted in the belief that the body holds the key to our deepest truths and inner wisdom, somatic education offers a unique approach to learning and growth—one that transcends traditional notions of intellectual knowledge and taps into the innate intelligence of the body. In this beginner's guide to somatic education, we will explore the foundational principles that underpin this transformative practice, offering insights and guidance for those who are embarking on this journey for the first time.

Embodied Learning: At the heart of somatic education lies the principle of embodied learning—a holistic approach to learning that integrates the body, mind, and spirit. Unlike traditional forms of education that prioritize intellectual knowledge and abstract concepts, embodied learning emphasizes direct experience and somatic awareness. Through somatic education, we learn not only with our minds but also with our bodies, engaging in experiential practices that deepen our understanding and insight.

Sensory Awareness: Central to somatic education is the cultivation of sensory awareness—the ability to tune into the subtle sensations and signals of the body. By developing greater sensory awareness, we can begin to unravel the mysteries of our own inner landscape, gaining insight into the patterns and habits that shape our thoughts, emotions, and behaviors. Through practices such as body scanning and mindful movement, we learn to listen to the wisdom of our bodies, allowing them to guide us on our journey of self-discovery.

Mind-Body Integration: Another key principle of somatic education is mind-body integration—the recognition that the mind and body are interconnected aspects of our being, each influencing and shaping the other in profound ways. Through somatic practices such as movement, breathwork, and mindfulness, we can cultivate greater harmony and alignment between our thoughts, emotions, and physical sensations, fostering a deeper sense of wholeness and well-being.

Experiential Learning: In somatic education, learning is not confined to the realm of intellectual understanding but is instead rooted in direct experience and embodied practice. Through experiential learning processes such as movement explorations, somatic exercises, and reflective inquiry, we engage in a process of discovery that is deeply personal and transformative. By immersing ourselves in the felt experience of our bodies, we can access deeper layers of insight and understanding, paving the way for profound growth and self-discovery.

Embodied Inquiry: Central to somatic education is the practice of embodied inquiry—a process of self-inquiry that is rooted in the body and its sensations. Through embodied inquiry, we explore questions such as "What am I feeling in this moment?" and "How does my body respond to different stimuli?" By approaching these questions with openness and curiosity, we can gain valuable insights into our own inner landscape, uncovering hidden truths and patterns that may have been obscured by habitual patterns of thought and behavior.

Holistic Approach: Somatic education takes a holistic approach to learning and growth, recognizing the interconnectedness of body, mind, and spirit. Rather than focusing solely on intellectual knowledge or physical skills, somatic education seeks to cultivate a deeper understanding of ourselves as integrated beings, honoring the wisdom of the body as a guide on our journey of self-discovery. By embracing this holistic perspective, we can tap into the full potential of our embodied experience, unlocking new realms of insight, creativity, and transformation.

By embracing embodied learning, sensory awareness, mind-body integration, experiential learning, embodied inquiry, and a holistic approach to learning and growth, we can embark on a journey of profound self-discovery and transformation, unlocking new realms of insight, creativity, and potential along the way.

1.3 Cultivating Body Awareness and Mindfulness

At the heart of this journey lies the cultivation of body awareness and mindfulness—a profound practice that invites us to deepen our connection to ourselves and the world around us. In this exploration of body awareness and mindfulness, we will delve into the foundational principles and practices that underpin this transformative journey, offering insights and guidance for those who seek to awaken to the fullness of their embodied experience.

Embodied Presence: Cultivating body awareness and mindfulness begins with the practice of embodied presence—a state of being fully awake and attuned to the present moment. In our fast-paced and often chaotic world, it can be easy to lose touch with our bodies and become disconnected from the richness of our sensory experience. Through somatic practices such as body scanning, mindful movement, and breath awareness, we can learn to anchor ourselves in the present moment, cultivating a deep sense of presence and aliveness in our bodies.

Sensory Exploration: Central to the practice of body awareness and mindfulness is the exploration of sensory experience—the rich tapestry of sensations that arise within the body from moment to moment. By tuning into the sensations of touch, proprioception, and interoception, we can begin to unravel the mysteries of our own inner landscape, gaining insight into the subtle nuances of our physical experience. Through practices such as body scans, mindful eating, and sensory awareness exercises, we can deepen our connection to our bodies and cultivate a more intimate relationship with ourselves.

Mindful Movement: Another key aspect of cultivating body awareness and mindfulness is the practice of mindful movement—an embodied practice that invites us to move with intention, awareness, and presence. Unlike traditional forms of exercise that focus solely on physical fitness, mindful movement emphasizes the quality of movement rather than the quantity, inviting us to explore the sensations, emotions, and intentions that arise as we move. Whether through practices such as yoga, tai chi, or somatic movement, mindful movement offers a powerful pathway to greater embodiment and self-awareness.

Breath Awareness: The breath serves as a powerful anchor for cultivating body awareness and mindfulness—a constant companion that accompanies us on our journey through life. By tuning into the rhythm of our breath, we can access a profound sense of presence and calm, grounding ourselves in the here and now. Through practices such as mindful breathing, breath observation, and breath-centered movement, we can harness the transformative power of the breath to deepen our connection to our bodies and cultivate greater mindfulness in our daily lives.

Interoceptive Awareness: Interoceptive awareness—the ability to perceive the sensations arising within the body—is a fundamental aspect of cultivating body awareness and mindfulness. By tuning into sensations such as hunger, thirst, and fatigue, we can gain valuable insight into our own physical and emotional well-being, learning to respond to the needs of our bodies with greater sensitivity and care. Through practices such as body scans, interoceptive awareness exercises, and mindful self-check-ins, we can deepen our connection to our bodies and cultivate a more compassionate relationship with ourselves.

Embodied Inquiry: Finally, cultivating body awareness and mindfulness is an ongoing process of inquiry—an exploration of the ever-changing landscape of our embodied experience. Through practices such as reflective journaling, body-based inquiry, and contemplative practices, we can deepen our understanding of ourselves and the world around us, gaining insight into the patterns, habits, and beliefs that shape our lives. By approaching this inquiry with openness, curiosity, and compassion, we can cultivate a deeper sense of self-awareness and presence, enriching our lives and relationships in profound and meaningful ways.

Cultivating body awareness and mindfulness is a transformative practice that invites us to awaken to the fullness of our embodied experience. By cultivating embodied presence, exploring sensory experience, engaging in mindful movement, tuning into the breath, developing interoceptive awareness, and embracing embodied inquiry, we can deepen our connection to ourselves and the world around us, fostering greater self-awareness, presence, and well-being in our lives.

1.4 Developing Interoception: Listening to Your Body's Signals

Interoception, the ability to perceive the subtle signals arising from within the body, is a skill that lies at the heart of somatic education. It is through the practice of interoception that we learn to listen to the whispers of our bodies, gaining insight into our physical and emotional well-being. In this exploration of interoception, we will delve into the intricacies of this profound practice, offering guidance and techniques for developing a deeper connection to our body's inner wisdom.

Embodied Awareness: Developing interoception begins with cultivating embodied awareness—an attunement to the sensations, feelings, and emotions that arise within the body from moment to moment. Rather than seeking to suppress or ignore these sensations, we learn to embrace them with curiosity and openness, recognizing them as valuable messengers guiding us on our journey of self-discovery. Through practices such as body scans, mindful movement, and breath awareness, we can deepen our connection to our bodies and cultivate a more intimate relationship with ourselves.

Tuning Into Sensations: Central to the practice of interoception is the art of tuning into sensations—the subtle cues and signals that emanate from within the body. By honing our ability to perceive sensations such as warmth, cold, pressure, and tension, we can gain valuable insight into our physical and emotional states, learning to respond to the needs of our bodies with greater sensitivity and care. Through practices such as body scans, sensory awareness exercises, and mindful self-check-ins, we can develop a more refined awareness of our body's inner landscape, enhancing our capacity for self-regulation and well-being.

Listening to Emotional Signals: In addition to physical sensations, interoception also encompasses the ability to perceive emotional signals arising within the body. Emotions, like physical sensations, manifest as subtle bodily sensations that can provide valuable insight into our emotional well-being. By learning to listen to these emotional signals with openness and curiosity, we can gain a deeper understanding of our emotional states, learning to respond to them with compassion and self-awareness. Through practices such as body-based inquiry, emotional check-ins, and contemplative practices, we can cultivate a more holistic awareness of ourselves, integrating the wisdom of both our bodies and our emotions into our lived experience.

Cultivating Self-Compassion: Developing interoception is not only about listening to our body's signals but also about responding to them with kindness and compassion. It is through the practice of self-compassion that we learn to meet our own needs with warmth and understanding, nurturing ourselves in times of distress and celebrating our successes with joy and appreciation. By cultivating a compassionate attitude towards ourselves and our bodies, we create a supportive inner environment that fosters growth, healing, and self-acceptance. Through practices such as loving-kindness meditation, self-soothing techniques, and compassionate self-talk, we can cultivate a more nurturing relationship with ourselves, laying the foundation for greater well-being and resilience.

Integration and Embodiment: Ultimately, the practice of interoception is about integration and embodiment—a deepening of our connection to ourselves and the world around us. It is through the integration of our physical, emotional, and cognitive experiences that we come to know ourselves more fully, embracing the totality of our human experience with openness and curiosity. By embodying the principles of interoception in our daily lives, we can cultivate a deeper sense of self-awareness, presence, and well-being, enriching our lives and relationships in profound and meaningful ways.

1.5 Preparing Your Mind and Environment for Somatic Practice

As we embark on the journey of somatic practice, it is essential to prepare both our minds and environments to create optimal conditions for growth, learning, and transformation. In this exploration, we will delve into the intricacies of preparing for somatic practice, offering guidance and insights to support you on your path to embodied well-being.

Cultivating a Beginner's Mind: Central to the preparation for somatic practice is the cultivation of a beginner's mind—an attitude of openness, curiosity, and receptivity to new experiences. Approaching each practice with a sense of wonder and exploration allows us to let go of preconceived notions and judgments, opening ourselves up to the richness of our inner landscape. By adopting a beginner's mind, we can cultivate a sense of humility and curiosity that invites us to learn and grow with each practice, embracing the journey of somatic exploration with enthusiasm and curiosity.

Creating a Sacred Space: Creating a sacred space for somatic practice is essential for fostering a sense of safety, comfort, and presence. Whether it's a dedicated yoga mat, a cozy corner of your home, or a serene outdoor setting, finding a space that resonates with you can enhance your practice and deepen your connection to yourself. By infusing your practice space with intention, beauty, and tranquility, you can create an environment that supports and nourishes your somatic journey, allowing you to immerse yourself fully in the present moment.

Setting Clear Intentions: Before beginning each somatic practice session, take a moment to set clear intentions for your practice. What do you hope to cultivate or explore during this session? Whether it's releasing tension, cultivating mindfulness, or deepening your body awareness, clarifying your intentions can help guide your practice and focus your attention. By setting clear intentions, you can align your practice with your goals and aspirations, harnessing the power of intention to support your growth and evolution on the mat and beyond.

Cultivating Mindfulness and Presence: Somatic practice invites us to cultivate mindfulness and presence—the art of being fully present and engaged in the unfolding moment. By cultivating mindfulness, we can deepen our awareness of our bodies, thoughts, and emotions, cultivating a sense of presence and aliveness that infuses every aspect of our lives. Whether it's through breath awareness, body scanning, or mindful movement, practicing mindfulness can help us become more attuned to the subtle nuances of our inner experience, fostering greater self-awareness and self-understanding.

Honoring Your Body's Wisdom: As you prepare for somatic practice, remember to honor your body's wisdom and listen to its cues and signals.

Your body is a wise and intelligent guide, offering valuable insights and feedback that can inform your practice and support your well-being. By listening to your body with compassion and curiosity, you can cultivate a deeper connection to yourself and develop a more harmonious relationship with your body. Trusting in your body's innate intelligence allows you to move with greater ease, grace, and authenticity, honoring the wisdom that resides within you.

Embracing the Journey: Finally, as you prepare for somatic practice, remember to embrace the journey with an open heart and mind. Somatic practice is not about achieving a specific outcome or mastering a particular technique—it's about the process of exploration, discovery, and self-inquiry. Allow yourself to be curious, playful, and adventurous as you navigate the landscape of your inner world, trusting in the wisdom of your body and the guidance of your intuition. Embrace the journey with humility, grace, and gratitude, knowing that each step you take brings you closer to a deeper understanding of yourself and the world around you.

ESSENTIAL SOMATIC EXERCISES FOR BEGINNERS

2.1 Gentle Somatic Movement: Basic Practices for Flexibility

Welcome to the world of gentle somatic movement—a realm where fluidity, ease, and flexibility reign supreme. In this chapter, we'll explore a variety of basic practices designed to enhance your flexibility and mobility, empowering you to move with greater freedom and grace. Whether you're brand new to somatic movement or a seasoned practitioner looking to deepen your practice, these gentle exercises offer a gateway to greater flexibility and well-being.

Before we dive into the specific exercises, let's take a moment to understand what gentle somatic movement is all about. Unlike traditional stretching or exercise routines, which often focus on forceful movements and external performance, gentle somatic movement emphasizes internal awareness, sensation, and exploration. By tuning into the subtle sensations of your body and moving with mindfulness and intention, you can cultivate greater flexibility, mobility, and ease in your movements.

The Cat-Cow Stretch

One of the most iconic and beneficial somatic movement exercises for flexibility is the Cat-Cow Stretch. To start, get on your hands and knees, placing your wrists exactly beneath your shoulders and your knees beneath your hips.. Breathe in, arching your back and pushing your chest up toward the ceiling while letting your belly fall to the ground. The cow position is this. Then, as you release the breath, draw your belly button toward your spine, round your spine, and tuck your chin into your chest. The

Cat position is this. As you move between these two positions, breathe in unison with your movements. The Cat-Cow Stretch gently mobilizes the spine, releases tension in the back and neck, and improves flexibility throughout the entire body.

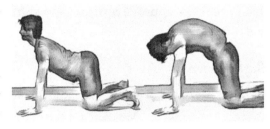

Forward Fold

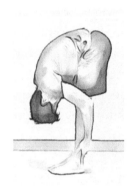

Another excellent somatic movement exercise for enhancing flexibility is the Forward Fold. Start by putting your feet hip-width apart and standing tall. As you exhale, hinge forward from your hips, allowing your torso to fold forward over your legs. Bend your knees as much as needed to maintain a comfortable stretch in the hamstrings and lower back. Let your head and neck relax, and allow your arms to hang loose toward the floor or hold onto opposite elbows for added support. Take several deep breaths in this position, feeling the stretch deepen with each exhale. The Forward Fold stretches the entire back body, including the spine, hamstrings, and calves, while also promoting relaxation and release.

The Shoulder Roll

For greater flexibility and mobility in the shoulders and upper back, try the Shoulder Roll exercise. Start by taking a tall stance and keeping your arms at your sides. Breathe in as you raise your shoulders to your ears, then release the air as you roll them back and forth in a fluid, circular motion. Continue this movement, focusing on releasing tension and increasing mobility in the shoulders. You can also reverse the direction of the shoulder roll, moving them forward and up on the inhale, and

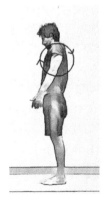

back and down on the exhale. The Shoulder Roll is an excellent way to relieve tension, improve posture, and enhance flexibility in the shoulders and upper back.

The Hip Opener

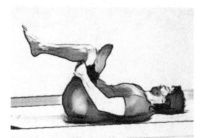

Consider attempting the Hip Opener exercise to improve hip suppleness and range of motion. Start by lying on your back with your feet flat on the ground and your knees bent. Form a figure-four with your legs by crossing your right ankle over your left knee. To protect your right knee, flex your right foot. Then, slowly press your right knee away from your body until your right hip and glute are stretched. After a few breaths, hold this position and switch sides. The Hip Opener stretches the hip rotators and glutes, helping to alleviate tightness and improve hip mobility.

The Spinal Twist

Another valuable somatic movement exercise for promoting flexibility is the Spinal Twist. Start by assuming a T-position while lying on your back with your arms out to the sides. Adjust your knees so that

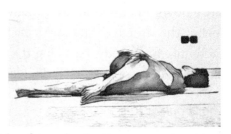

they are bent and rest on the right side of your body. Keep your shoulders grounded as you gently rotate your torso to the left, bringing your left knee toward the floor. You can place your right hand on your left knee to deepen the stretch if desired. Hold this position for several breaths, feeling the twist gently unravel tension in the spine and promote flexibility in the torso. Then, switch sides and repeat the movement. The Spinal Twist helps to release stiffness in the spine, increase mobility in the thoracic region, and improve overall spinal health.

The Seated Forward Bend

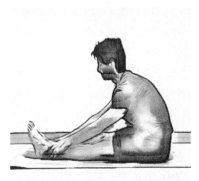

For a gentle yet effective stretch for the hamstrings and lower back, try the Seated Forward Bend. Starting from the floor, sit with your legs straight out in front of you. Flex your feet inward toward your body while sitting up straight and elongating your spine. Lean forward from your hips and extend your hands toward your shins or feet as you release the breath. Bend forward, letting your head drop to your knees, maintaining a long spine and an open chest. As you hold this position for a few deep breaths, feel the stretch getting deeper with each exhale. The Seated Forward Bend releases tension in the hamstrings, calves, and lower back, while also calming the mind and promoting relaxation.

The Standing Side Stretch

To increase flexibility in the sides of the body and promote greater mobility in the spine, try the Standing Side Stretch. Step one: Take a tall stance, place your feet hip-width apart, and keep your arms at your sides. Take a breath and extend your arms overhead, folding your fingers together and pressing your palms up against the ceiling. Exhale as you lean gently to one side, creating a long line of energy from your fingertips down to your feet. Keep both feet grounded as you lengthen through the sides of 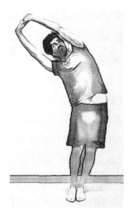 your body and open up the ribcage. Hold this stretch for several breaths, then return to center and repeat on the other side. The Standing Side Stretch stretches the intercostal muscles between the ribs, promotes spinal flexibility, and encourages deep breathing.

The Quadriceps Stretch

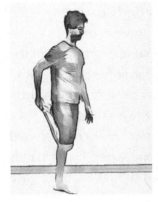

For greater flexibility and mobility in the quadriceps muscles, try the Quadriceps Stretch. Start by putting your feet hip-width apart and standing tall. By bending your right knee and shifting your weight to your left foot, you can bring your right heel closer to your glutes. Reach back with your right hand and gently grasp your right ankle or shin, bringing your heel closer to your body. Keep your knees close together and your pelvis neutral as you feel the stretch in the front of your right thigh. Hold this position for several breaths, then switch sides and repeat the stretch on the left leg. The Quadriceps Stretch helps to release tension in the front of the thighs, improve hip flexor mobility, and enhance overall lower body flexibility.

The Chest Opener

To release tension in the chest and shoulders and promote better posture, try the Chest Opener somatic movement. Begin by standing tall with your feet hip-width apart and your arms relaxed at your sides. Inhale deeply as you reach your arms behind you, interlacing your fingers and squeezing your shoulder blades together. Lift your chest and gaze upward slightly to deepen the stretch in the front of your body. Hold this position for a few breaths, feeling the expansion

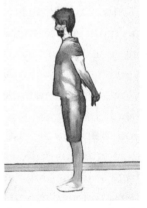

across the chest and shoulders. Exhale as you release your arms back down to your sides. The Chest Opener helps counteract the forward slump often associated with prolonged sitting or computer work, improving posture and opening the heart center.

The Supine Leg Stretch

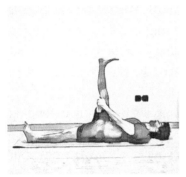

To increase flexibility in the hamstrings and improve mobility in the hips, try the Supine Leg Stretch. Start by lying on your back with your feet flat on the ground and your knees bent. Extend your right leg straight up toward the ceiling, flexing your foot to engage the muscles of the leg. Hold the back of your thigh with both hands, or loop a strap around your foot if you need additional support. Keep your left leg bent or extend it along the floor for a deeper stretch. Hold this position for several breaths, feeling the lengthening sensation in the back of your right leg. Then, switch legs and repeat the stretch on the left side. The Supine Leg Stretch helps to release tightness in the hamstrings, increase flexibility in the hips, and improve overall lower body mobility.

2.2 Introduction to Pandiculation: Techniques for Relaxation

Pandiculation is a powerful yet gentle practice that can profoundly impact our physical and mental well-being. In this section, we will explore the fundamentals of pandiculation, its benefits, and how to incorporate it into your somatic practice for deep relaxation and tension relief.

Understanding Pandiculation

Pandiculation is a natural movement pattern found in many animals, including humans. It involves three distinct phases: contraction, elongation, and relaxation. During the contraction phase, muscles are gently contracted or tightened, activating sensory receptors known as proprioceptors. These receptors send signals to the brain, informing it of the current state of muscle tension and length.

The Process of Pandiculation

To perform a pandiculation, begin by consciously contracting a specific muscle or muscle group. For example, you might contract your **hamstrings** by gently bending your knees and pulling your heels towards your buttocks. Hold this contraction for a few seconds, allowing yourself to feel the tension in the muscles.

Next, slowly and deliberately lengthen the muscles by gently extending the limbs or moving the body in the opposite direction. For instance, you could slowly straighten your legs and reach your heels away from your body, feeling the stretch in your **hamstrings**. This elongation phase helps to reset the muscle length and improve flexibility.

Finally, allow the muscles to relax completely, releasing any residual tension or tightness. Focus on breathing deeply and consciously, allowing the breath to facilitate the release of tension throughout the body. As you relax, notice any changes in sensation or perception, such as increased warmth or a sense of heaviness in the muscles.

Benefits of Pandiculation

Pandiculation offers numerous benefits for both the body and mind. By actively engaging with the muscles and sensory feedback, pandiculation helps to improve proprioception, or the body's awareness of its position in space. This increased proprioceptive awareness can enhance movement efficiency, coordination, and balance.

Additionally, pandiculation promotes relaxation by encouraging the release of stored tension and stress in the muscles. As you engage in the contraction, elongation, and relaxation phases, you may notice a profound sense of ease and comfort spreading throughout your body. This relaxation response can help to reduce muscle soreness, alleviate stiffness, and promote a greater sense of overall well-being.

Incorporating Pandiculation into Your Practice

To incorporate pandiculation into your somatic practice, start by focusing on specific muscle groups or areas of tension in the body. Experiment with different movements and positions to target areas that feel tight or restricted. For example, you might practice pandiculating your **neck** and **shoulders** to release tension from hours of sitting at a desk.

As you become more familiar with pandiculation, you can gradually expand your practice to include full-body movements and sequences. Remember to move slowly and mindfully, paying attention to the sensations and feedback from your body. Honor your body's limits and avoid pushing into pain or discomfort.

2.3 Dynamic Somatic Movements for Strength and Stability

Dynamic somatic movements are an essential component of any somatic practice, offering a unique opportunity to build strength, stability, and mobility in the body. In this section, we will explore the principles of dynamic somatic movements, their benefits, and how to incorporate them into your practice for optimal results.

Understanding Dynamic Somatic Movements

Dynamic somatic movements involve fluid, continuous movements that engage multiple muscle groups and joints simultaneously. Unlike static stretches or isolated exercises, dynamic movements emphasize functional movement patterns that mimic real-life activities. By moving dynamically, we can improve coordination, proprioception, and overall movement efficiency.

The Benefits of Dynamic Movements

Dynamic somatic movements offer a wide range of benefits for both physical and mental well-being. From increased flexibility and joint mobility to enhanced muscular strength and endurance, dynamic movements provide a comprehensive workout for the entire body. Additionally, dynamic movements promote greater body awareness and mindfulness, helping to improve concentration and focus.

Incorporating Dynamic Movements into Your Practice

To incorporate dynamic movements into your somatic practice, start by warming up the body with gentle movements such as **dynamic shoulder circles** and **hip circles**. These movements help to lubricate the joints, increase blood flow, and prepare the body for more vigorous activity.

Once warmed up, progress to more challenging dynamic movements that target specific areas of the body. For example, you might perform **dynamic lunges** to strengthen the legs and improve balance, or **dynamic spinal twists** to mobilize the spine and improve flexibility. Remember to move with intention and awareness, paying attention to how each movement feels in your body.

As you become more comfortable with dynamic movements, you can begin to incorporate them into full-body sequences and routines. Experiment with different combinations of movements to create a dynamic flow that addresses your unique needs and goals. Whether you're looking to improve athletic performance, enhance functional movement, or simply feel better in your body, dynamic somatic movements offer a versatile and effective approach to fitness and well-being.

Sample Dynamic Somatic Movements

1. Dynamic Shoulder Circles

Stand tall with your feet hip-width apart. Begin by circling your shoulders forward in a smooth, continuous motion. As you circle your shoulders, focus on engaging the muscles of your upper back and chest. After several repetitions, reverse the direction of the circles, this time circling your shoulders backward.

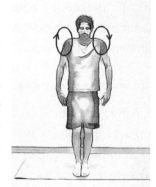

2. Dynamic Hip Circles

Stand with your feet hip-width apart and your hands on your hips. Begin by circling your hips in a clockwise direction, making smooth, controlled movements. As you circle your hips, focus on maintaining stability in your core and pelvis. After several repetitions, reverse the direction of the circles, this time circling your hips counterclockwise.

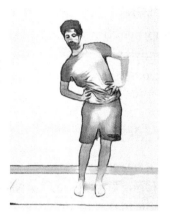

3. Dynamic Lunges

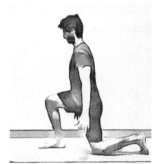

Place your feet together and stand at the beginning. Taking a step with your right foot, lower your body into a lunge. Maintain the alignment of your front knee with your ankle and the slight elevation of your back knee as you lunge. Repeat on the other side after pushing off your front foot to get back to the starting position.

4. Dynamic Spinal Twists

Place your legs out in front of you while sitting on the floor. Position your right foot outside of your left knee while bending your right knee. For support, place your right hand behind you and your left hand on your right knee. Breathe in to lengthen your spine; then, as you twist to the right, gently move your right knee across your body with 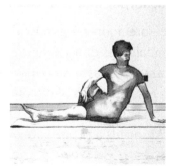 your left hand while exhaling. After a few breaths of holding, go back to the beginning and repeat on the other side.

By incorporating dynamic movements into your somatic practice, you can improve coordination, flexibility, and overall physical fitness. Start exploring dynamic movements today and experience the transformative power of mindful movement.

2.4 Exploring Muscle Release Patterns: Releasing Tension

Muscle release patterns are a fundamental aspect of somatic movement, offering a pathway to release tension and promote relaxation in the body. In this section, we will delve into the intricate patterns of muscular tension and how to effectively release tension through somatic techniques. By understanding these patterns and practicing targeted exercises, you can experience greater ease and freedom in your body.

Understanding Muscle Tension Patterns

Muscle tension patterns refer to the habitual ways in which muscles contract and hold tension in response to stress, injury, or poor movement habits. These patterns often develop unconsciously over time and can lead to discomfort, pain, and limited range of motion. The neck, shoulders, lower back, hips, and jaw are frequently tense spots.

Identifying Muscle Imbalances

Before addressing muscle tension patterns, it's essential to identify any imbalances or asymmetries in the body. This can be done through a process of self-assessment, where you observe your posture, movement patterns, and areas of discomfort or restriction. By pinpointing areas of tension and imbalance, you can tailor your somatic practice to address specific needs and promote overall balance and alignment.

Techniques for Releasing Muscle Tension

Once you've identified areas of tension, you can begin to explore techniques for releasing muscle tension and promoting relaxation. One effective technique is **contract-relax**, where you intentionally contract a muscle group before releasing it to encourage relaxation and lengthening. For example, you might contract your **quadriceps** by pressing your knee into the floor, then release and feel the muscles soften and lengthen.

Another effective technique is **self-massage**, where you use your hands or a massage tool to apply pressure to tense or tight areas. This may aid in promoting relaxation, lowering muscle soreness, and increasing blood flow. Focus on areas of tension such as the **trapezius muscles** in the shoulders or the **gluteal muscles** in the hips, using gentle pressure and circular motions to release tension.

Exploring Specific Muscle Release Exercises

To target specific muscle release patterns, incorporate exercises that focus on stretching and lengthening tight muscles. For example, the **cat-cow stretch** is an excellent exercise for releasing tension in the spine and promoting flexibility. Begin on your hands and knees, arching your back up towards the ceiling as you exhale (cat pose), then lowering your belly towards the floor as you inhale (cow pose).

Another effective exercise is the **hip flexor stretch**, which targets tightness in the hip flexors and psoas muscles. Start in a kneeling position with one foot forward, pressing your hips forward until you feel a stretch in the front of your hip. Hold for several breaths, then switch sides to stretch the opposite hip flexor.

Incorporating Mindfulness and Breathwork

In addition to physical exercises, incorporating mindfulness and breathwork can enhance the effectiveness of muscle release techniques. By bringing awareness to your breath and focusing on the present moment, you can cultivate a sense of relaxation and ease in both body and mind. Practice deep, diaphragmatic breathing as you perform muscle release exercises, allowing your breath to guide you deeper into relaxation.

Exploring muscle release patterns and techniques is an essential aspect of somatic movement, offering a pathway to release tension, promote relaxation, and improve overall well-being.

TARGETED SOMATIC EXERCISES
FOR COMMON ISSUES

3.1 Neck and Shoulder Release Techniques for Beginners

Before delving into specific techniques, it's essential to understand the root causes of neck and shoulder tension. Poor posture, repetitive movements, and emotional stress can all contribute to tightness in this area. Additionally, modern lifestyles that involve prolonged periods of sitting and sedentary behavior can exacerbate tension in the neck and shoulders.

The Importance of Relaxation

One of the key principles of releasing tension in the neck and shoulders is relaxation. When we're stressed or tense, our muscles tend to contract and hold tension, leading to discomfort and stiffness. By practicing relaxation techniques, we can encourage the muscles to soften and release, promoting greater ease and comfort in the neck and shoulders.

Gentle Neck Stretches

The neck is a complex and delicate area of the body that is prone to tension and stiffness, especially in today's sedentary lifestyles. Gentle neck stretches are essential for relieving tightness, improving flexibility, and promoting relaxation in the neck muscles. In this section, we will explore various gentle neck stretches that beginners can incorporate into their daily routine.

1. Side Neck Stretch

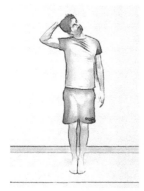

Begin by sitting or standing tall with your spine straight and shoulders relaxed. Gently tilt your head to one side, bringing your ear towards your shoulder until you feel a stretch along the side of your neck. Avoid lifting your shoulder towards your ear; instead, keep it relaxed and away from your ear. Maintain this posture for 15–30 seconds while taking slow, deep breaths. Sensationally stretch the sternocleidomastoid muscle on the side of your neck. Repeat on the opposite side.

2. Forward Neck Stretch

Interlace your fingers and place your hands be-hind your head. Gently press your head forward with your hands, allowing your chin to move to-wards your chest. Keep your shoulders relaxed and avoid hunching them towards your ears. You should feel a gentle stretch along the back of your neck and between your shoulder blades. Breathe slowly and deeply as you hold this posi-

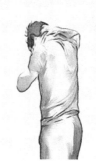

tion for 15 to 30 seconds. This stretch is intended to work the levator scap-ulae and upper trapezius muscles.

3. Chin to Chest Stretch

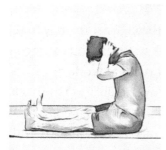

Feel the back of your neck stretch as you slouch and slowly bring your chin up to your chest. Keep your shoulders relaxed and avoid rounding your upper back excessively. Hold this position for 15-30 seconds, breathing deeply and allowing the muscles in the back of your neck to release. This stretch helps re-lieve tension in the **suboccipital** muscles and promotes flexibility in the neck.

4. Rotation Neck Stretch

Begin by taking a tall stance or sitting with your shoulders relaxed and your spine straight. Bring your chin up to your shoulder as you slowly turn your head to one side. Keep your gaze forward and avoid lifting or dropping your chin excessively. You should feel a gentle stretch along the side of your neck and into your upper back. Hold this position for 15-30 seconds, breathing deeply and allowing the muscles to relax. Repeat on the opposite side. This stretch targets the **levator scapulae** and **scalene** muscles.

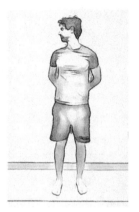

5. Ear to Shoulder Stretch

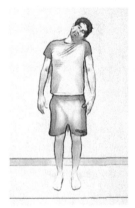

Start by taking a tall stance or sitting with your shoulders relaxed and your spine straight. Bring your ear close to your shoulder as you gently cock your head to one side. Avoid lifting your shoulder towards your ear; instead, keep it relaxed and away from your ear. You should feel a stretch along the side of your neck. Hold this position for 15-30 seconds while breathing deeply and slowly. Repeat on the opposite side. This stretch targets the **trapezius** and **levator scapulae** muscles.

Incorporating Gentle Neck Stretches into Your Routine

These gentle neck stretches can be performed throughout the day to relieve tension and promote relaxation in the neck muscles. You can incorporate them into your morning routine, during breaks at work, or before bed to help release accumulated stress and improve flexibility in the neck. Remember to perform each stretch slowly and gently, listening to your body and avoiding any movements that cause pain or discomfort. With consistent practice, you can enjoy greater ease and comfort in your neck and shoulders, leading to improved overall well-being.

Shoulder Rolls and Releases

Shoulder rolls and releases are fundamental movements for promoting mobility, relaxation, and tension relief in the shoulders and upper back. In this section, we will explore various techniques and exercises to perform shoulder rolls and releases effectively.

1. Shoulder Roll Technique

Start by standing tall with your feet hip-width apart and your arms relaxed by your sides. Begin to roll your shoulders forward in a circular motion, moving them up towards your ears, then back and down, and finally forward again. Focus on making the movement smooth and fluid, allowing your shoulder blades to glide along your back. Perform 5-10 forward shoulder rolls, then reverse the motion and perform 5-10 backward shoulder rolls.

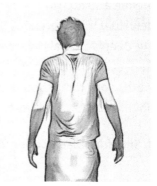

2. Shoulder Circle Exercise

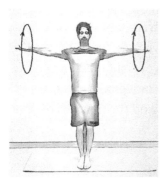

Stand with your feet hip-width apart and your arms relaxed by your sides. Extend your arms out to the sides at shoulder height, forming a T-shape with your body. Begin to make small circles with your shoulders, moving them forward in a circular motion. Focus on keeping your neck relaxed and your movements controlled. Gradually increase the size of the circles, making them as large as feels comfortable. After 10-15 forward circles, reverse the motion and perform 10-15 backward circles.

3. Shoulder Release Stretch

Stand tall with your feet hip-width apart and your arms relaxed by your sides. Reach your right arm across your chest towards your left shoulder, placing your hand on the top of your left shoulder. Use your left hand to gently press your right elbow towards your chest, feeling a stretch in the back of your right shoulder. Hold this stretch for 15-30 seconds, breathing deeply and allowing the muscles to relax.

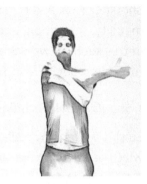

Repeat on the opposite side, reaching your left arm across your chest towards your right shoulder and using your right hand to press your left elbow towards your chest.

4. Shoulder Blade Squeeze

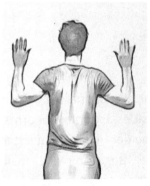

With your shoulders relaxed and your spine straight, sit or stand tall. Starting from the back, squeeze your shoulder blades together as though you were attempting to hold a pencil between them. Feel the muscles between your shoulder blades contract as you hold the squeeze for three to five seconds. Let go of the pressure and permit your shoulder blades to separate. Repeat this movement 10-15 times, focusing on maintaining good posture and engaging the muscles of your upper back.

5. Arm Circles

Stand with your feet hip-width apart and your arms extended out to the sides at shoulder height. Begin to make small circles with your arms, moving them forward in a circular motion. Focus on keeping your shoulders re-

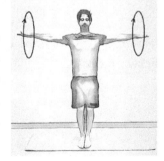

laxed and your movements controlled. Gradually increase the size of the circles, making them as large as feels comfortable. After 10-15 forward circles, reverse the motion and perform 10-15 backward circles.

Incorporating Shoulder Rolls and Releases into Your Routine

Shoulder rolls and releases can be performed as part of your warm-up routine before exercise, as a midday break to release tension, or as part of your evening relaxation practice. These movements are effective for relieving stiffness and promoting mobility in the shoulders and upper back. Practice them regularly to maintain healthy shoulder function and prevent discomfort and injury. Remember to listen to your body and adjust the intensity of the movements as needed to suit your level of flexibility and comfort.

Incorporating Breathwork and Mindfulness

As you practice these neck and shoulder release techniques, remember to focus on your breath and cultivate a sense of mindfulness. Breathe deeply into the areas of tension, allowing your breath to guide you deeper into relaxation. Notice any sensations that arise in the body, and practice letting go of tension with each exhale. By combining breathwork and mindfulness with targeted stretching exercises, you can enhance the effectiveness of your practice and promote greater ease and comfort in the neck and shoulders.

3.2 Hip and Lower Back Mobility Exercises

Hip and lower back mobility exercises are essential for maintaining flexibility, reducing stiffness, and preventing discomfort in these areas. In this section, we will explore a variety of practical exercises and techniques to improve hip and lower back mobility.

1. Pelvic Tilts

Pelvic tilts are an effective exercise for mobilizing the lower back and pelvis.

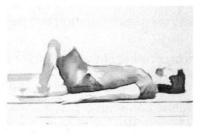

How to Perform Pelvic Tilts:
- With your feet flat on the ground and your knees bent, lie on your back.
- Place your hands on your hips or by your sides for support.
- Inhale to prepare, then exhale as you gently tilt your pelvis backward, flattening your lower back against the floor.
- Hold the position for a few seconds, then inhale as you return to the starting position.
- Repeat for 10-15 repetitions, focusing on the smooth movement of the pelvis.

2. Figure-Four Stretch

The figure-four stretch targets the hips and glutes, promoting flexibility and mobility in these areas.

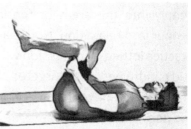

How to Perform the Figure-Four Stretch:
- With your feet flat on the ground and your knees bent, lie on your back.
- Cross your right ankle over your left knee, forming a figure-four shape with your legs.
- Reach your hands around your left thigh and gently pull your left knee towards your chest until you feel a stretch in your right hip and glute.
- Hold the stretch for 15-30 seconds, breathing deeply and relaxing into the stretch.
- Repeat on the opposite side, crossing your left ankle over your right knee and pulling your right knee towards your chest.

3. Cat-Cow Stretch

The cat-cow stretch is a dynamic movement that targets the entire spine, including the lower back and hips.

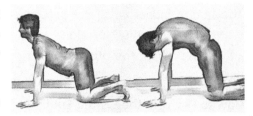

How to Perform the Cat-Cow Stretch:
- Start on your hands and knees in a tabletop position, with your wrists aligned under your shoulders and your knees under your hips.
- Inhale as you arch your back, lowering your belly towards the floor and lifting your head and tailbone towards the ceiling (cow pose).
- Breathe out as you round your back, bringing your navel toward your spine and tucking your chin into your chest (cat pose).
- Continue flowing between cow and cat poses, coordinating your breath with your movement.
- Repeat for 10-15 repetitions, focusing on the fluidity of the spine.

4. Hip Flexor Stretch

The hip flexor stretch targets the muscles at the front of the hip, promoting flexibility and mobility in this area.

How to Perform the Hip Flexor Stretch:
- Move your weight forward a little bit until your right hip's front starts to stretch.
- Shift your weight forward slightly until you feel a stretch in the front of your right hip.
- To stay stable, keep your torso straight and contract your core..
- Hold the stretch for 15-30 seconds, then switch sides and repeat on the opposite leg.

5. Seated Spinal Twist:

The seated spinal twist is a seated pose that targets the muscles along the spine and in the hips, promoting flexibility and mobility.

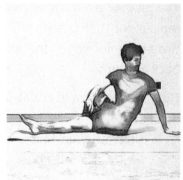

How to Perform the Seated Spinal Twist:
- Sit on the floor with your legs extended in front of you.
- Bend your right knee and cross it over your left leg, placing your right foot flat on the floor next to your left thigh.
- As you twist your torso to the right and place your left elbow on the outside of your right knee, take a breath to lengthen your spine and release it.
- Use your right hand for support behind you, pressing into the floor to deepen the twist.
- Hold the stretch for 15-30 seconds, then switch sides and repeat on the opposite side.

Incorporating Hip and Lower Back Mobility Exercises into Your Routine

These exercises can be incorporated into your daily routine to improve hip and lower back mobility. Perform them regularly to maintain flexibility, reduce stiffness, and prevent discomfort in these areas. Remember to listen to your body and modify the exercises as needed to suit your level of flexibility and comfort.

3.3 Spine Alignment Practices for Posture Improvement

Spine alignment practices are crucial for maintaining good posture and preventing discomfort or pain associated with poor spinal alignment. In this section, we will explore a series of practical exercises and techniques designed to improve spine alignment for better posture.

1. Mountain Pose (Tadasana)

Mountain pose is a foundational yoga posture that helps align the spine and promote proper posture.

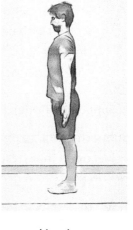

How to Perform Mountain Pose:

- Stand tall with your feet hip-width apart, distributing your weight evenly on both feet.
- Engage your leg muscles and lift your knee-caps, drawing your thighs back slightly.
- Lengthen your tailbone towards the floor and engage your core muscles.
- Open your chest by rolling your shoulders down and back.
- With your palms facing forward, extend your arms out in front of you.
- Relax your neck and gaze forward, keeping your chin parallel to the floor.
- Hold the pose for 30 seconds to 1 minute, focusing on elongating the spine and maintaining proper alignment.

2. Forward Fold (Uttanasana)

Forward fold is a yoga pose that stretches the spine, hamstrings, and calves while promoting spinal elongation and alignment.

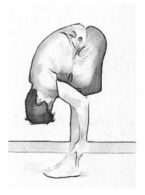

How to Perform Forward Fold:

- Start in a standing position with your feet hip-width apart.
- Exhale as you hinge at the hips and fold forward, keeping your spine long.
- Bend your knees slightly if necessary to maintain a straight spine.
- Let your neck and head fall back toward the floor.

- Hold onto your elbows with opposite hands or place your hands on the floor or blocks for support.
- Lengthen through your spine with each inhale and deepen the stretch with each exhale.
- Hold the pose for 30 seconds to 1 minute, breathing deeply and focusing on spinal alignment.

3. Supported Bridge Pose

Supported bridge pose helps align the spine, open the chest, and release tension in the back muscles.

How to Perform Supported Bridge Pose:

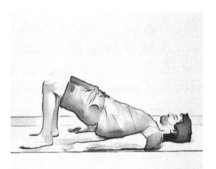

- Lie on your back with your knees bent and feet hip-width apart, heels close to your buttocks.
- Place a yoga block or folded blanket under your sacrum for support.
- Press into your feet and lift your hips towards the ceiling, engaging your glutes and core.
- Keep your chin slightly tucked to maintain a neutral spine and avoid straining your neck.
- Hold the pose for 30 seconds to 1 minute, focusing on lengthening the spine and opening the chest.
- Slowly lower your hips back down to the floor and remove the prop.

4. Standing Forward Bend with Shoulder Opener

This variation of the standing forward bend incorporates a shoulder opener to enhance spinal alignment and posture.

How to Perform Standing Forward Bend with Shoulder Opener:

- Stand with your feet hip-width apart and interlace your fingers behind your back.

- Inhale to lengthen your spine, then exhale as you fold forward at the hips, bringing your arms overhead.
- Allow your head and neck to relax towards the floor and keep a slight bend in your knees if needed.
- Feel the stretch in your hamstrings, spine, and shoulders.
- Hold the pose for 30 seconds to 1 minute, breathing deeply and focusing on spinal elongation.
- To release, gently release your hands to the floor and slowly roll up to standing.

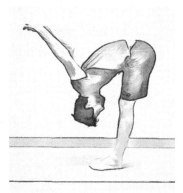

Incorporating Spine Alignment Practices into Your Routine

These exercises can be incorporated into your daily routine to improve spine alignment and posture. Practice them regularly to strengthen the muscles that support your spine, release tension, and maintain optimal spinal alignment for overall health and well-being. Remember to listen to your body and modify the exercises as needed to suit your individual needs and abilities.

3.4 Hands, Feet, and Joint Mobilization Basics

In this section, we'll delve into fundamental exercises and techniques to mobilize the hands, feet, and joints, essential for improving flexibility, mobility, and overall well-being.

1. Hand Mobilization Exercises

Hand mobilization exercises are beneficial for maintaining dexterity, relieving stiffness, and preventing discomfort in the hands and wrists.

Finger Flexion and Extension:
- Sit or stand comfortably with your hands resting on a flat surface.

- Slowly curl your fingers into a fist, squeezing gently, then extend them fully, spreading them apart.
- Repeat this movement 10-15 times, focusing on the full range of motion in your fingers and joints.

Wrist Circles:
- Extend your arms in front of you at shoulder height, palms facing down.
- Start turning your wrists in a clockwise and then counterclockwise direction.
- Perform 10-15 rotations in each direction, keeping the movements smooth and controlled.

2. Foot Mobilization Exercises

Foot mobilization exercises help improve balance, flexibility, and mobility in the feet and ankles.

Toe Flex and Point:
- Sit on a chair with your feet flat on the floor.
- Slowly flex your toes towards the soles of your feet, then point them away, stretching the tops of your feet.
- Repeat this movement 10-15 times, focusing on the articulation of each toe.

Ankle Circles:
- Sit or lie down with your legs extended in front of you.
- Make a clockwise and counterclockwise rotation with your ankles.
- Perform 10-15 rotations in each direction, keeping the movements fluid and controlled.

3. Joint Mobilization Techniques

Joint mobilization techniques help increase the range of motion, reduce stiffness, and promote joint health.

Shoulder Rolls:
- Stand tall with your arms relaxed by your sides.

- Breathe in as you raise your shoulders to your ears; as you lower them back down, breathe out.
- Repeat this motion 10-15 times, focusing on smooth, controlled movements and relaxation of the shoulder muscles.

Hip Circles:
- Stand with your feet hip-width apart and hands on your hips.
- Start rotating your hips in a clockwise and counterclockwise direction.
- Perform 10-15 rotations in each direction, focusing on the mobility of your hip joints.

4. Integration Exercises

Integration exercises combine movements of the hands, feet, and joints to improve coordination and overall mobility.

Hand-to-Foot Coordination:
- Sit on the floor with your legs extended in front of you.
- Reach your right hand towards your left foot, crossing your body diagonally.
- Return to the starting position and repeat on the opposite side.

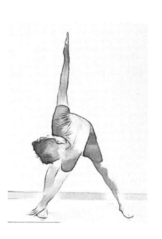

- Continue alternating sides for 10-15 repetitions, focusing on smooth, coordinated movements.

Full Body Circles:
- Stand with your feet hip-width apart and arms extended out to the sides.
- Begin to circle your arms overhead as you rise up onto your toes.
- Lower your arms and heels as you circle them back down to the starting position.
- Repeat this motion for 10-15 repetitions, focusing on the integration of movement throughout your entire body.

Incorporate these hands, feet, and joint mobilization basics into your daily routine to enhance flexibility, mobility, and overall joint health. Practice regularly and pay attention to how your body responds, making adjustments as needed to suit your individual needs and abilities.

MASTERING SOMATIC MOVEMENT: 4 ESSENTIAL EXERCISE ROUTINES FOR BALANCE AND WELL-BEING

4.1 Routine 1: Foundational Somatic Flow

Duration: 20 minutes

1. **Somatic Body Scan:** Start by lying comfortably on your back, arms by your sides, and legs extended. Close your eyes and bring awareness to each part of your body, from your head to your toes, releasing tension as you go. Take slow, deep breaths as you scan through your body.

2. **Pandiculation of Major Muscle Groups:** From a standing position, begin with the neck and shoulders, gently contracting and releasing the muscles. Move down to the spine, arching and rounding the back. Then, focus on the hips and legs, bending and straightening the knees. Repeat this sequence three times, allowing for fluid movement and relaxation.

3. **Somatic Cat-Cow Stretch:** Come to a tabletop position on your hands and knees. Take a breath and raise your tailbone and chest toward the ceiling by arching your back (cow pose). Pull your chin in toward your chest and release the breath as you round your spine (cat pose). Perform five rounds of these two poses while breathing.

4. **Somatic Side Bend:** Sit cross-legged on the floor or in a chair. Inhale as you reach your right arm overhead, lengthening through the side body. Exhale and gently lean to the left, feeling the

stretch along the right side. After a few breaths of holding, switch sides. On each side, repeat three times.

5. **Somatic Leg Swing**: Position your feet hip-width apart. Should you require assistance, cling to a sturdy object. With deliberate movement, swing your right leg forward and backward, sensing the movement coming from your hip joint.Swing for 10 repetitions, then switch to the left leg.

6. **Full-Body Shake**: Stand with feet shoulder-width apart and shake your arms, legs, and torso gently for 1 minute. Let go of any remaining tension as you allow your body to shake freely.

7. **Final Relaxation**: Lie down on your back in Savasana (Corpse Pose). Allow your body to completely relax as you close your eyes and concentrate on your breathing. Take five to ten minutes to rest here and absorb the advantages of your practice.

4.2 Routine 2: Targeted Somatic Release

Duration: 15 minutes

1. **Neck and Shoulder Release**: Sit comfortably in a chair or on the floor. Gently press your right ear against your right shoulder until you feel a stretch on the left side of your neck. Exchange sides after a few breaths of holding. Proceed three times on every side.

2. **Spinal Twist**: Sit cross-legged on the floor or in a chair. Inhale to lengthen your spine, then exhale as you twist to the right, placing your left hand on your right knee and your right hand behind you for support. Hold for 5 breaths, then repeat on the opposite side.

3. **Hip Opener**: With your feet flat on the ground and your knees bent, lie on your back. Flex your right foot by crossing your right ankle over your left knee. Clasp your hands behind your left thigh and pass your right arm through the opening between your legs. You should feel a stretch in your right hip as you bring your left knee up to your chest. After five breaths of holding, switch sides.

4. **Forward Fold**: Position your feet hip-width apart. Breathe in to extend your back and out as you fold forward, bending your

knees slightly, while hunching forward at the hips. Turn your head and neck in the direction of the floor. After holding for five breaths, gradually rise to your feet.

5. **Somatic Foot Release**: Sit on the floor with legs extended. Flex and point your toes several times, then rotate your ankles in both directions. Massage the soles of your feet with your hands, paying attention to any areas of tension.

6. **Breath Awareness**: Close your eyes and bring your attention to your breath. Notice the rise and fall of your chest and the sensation of air entering and leaving your nostrils. Take slow, deep breaths, allowing each exhale to release stress and tension.

7. **Final Relaxation**: Lie down on your back in Savasana (Corpse Pose) with arms by your sides and palms facing up. Relax your entire body, allowing the floor to support you fully. Stay here for 5-10 minutes, breathing deeply and surrendering to the present moment.

4.3 Routine 3: Somatic Mobility Sequence

Duration: 25 minutes

1. **Somatic Breathwork**: Begin in a comfortable seated position. Close your eyes and take a few deep breaths, focusing on the sensation of the breath moving in and out of your body. Allow your breath to become slow and steady.

2. **Neck Release**: Sit tall with your spine elongated. Drop your chin towards your chest and slowly roll your head to the right, then back to center, and to the left. Repeat this movement 5 times in each direction, allowing the neck muscles to release tension.

3. **Shoulder Rolls**: When you inhale, raise your shoulders toward your ears, and when you exhale, lower them again. Repeat this shoulder roll motion 8-10 times, focusing on opening up the chest and releasing tightness in the shoulders.

4. **Spinal Wave**: Take a cross-legged seat in a chair or on the floor. Take a breath, arch your back, lift your chest, and look up at the

ceiling. Tuck your chin into your chest and release the breath as you round your spine. Flow smoothly between these two movements, creating a wave-like motion through your spine. Repeat for 5 rounds.

5. **Hip Circles**: With your feet flat on the ground, take a seat on a chair's edge. Place your hands on your knees and gently circle your hips clockwise for 8 repetitions, then reverse the direction for another 8 repetitions. Focus on creating smooth and controlled movements.

6. **Dynamic Forward Fold**: Position your feet hip-width apart. Breathe in while extending your arms overhead and lengthening your spine. Let out a breath as you extend your hands toward your shins or the ground while hunching forward from your hips. To return to a standing position, inhale. For eight to ten repetitions, perform this dynamic forward fold while matching your breathing to your movements.

7. **Seated Twist**: Sit cross-legged on the floor or in a chair. Inhale to lengthen your spine, then exhale as you twist to the right, placing your left hand on your right knee and your right hand behind you for support. After a short period of holding, move back to the center and repeat on the left side. For three rounds, switch between the two sides.

8. **Standing Side Stretch**: Stand with feet hip-width apart. Inhale as you reach your right arm overhead, stretching through the right side of your body. Hold for a few breaths, then switch to the left side. Repeat this side stretch movement 5 times on each side, focusing on elongating the side body.

9. **Final Relaxation**: Lie down on your back in Savasana (Corpse Pose). Let your body sink fully into the floor while you close your eyes. With each exhale, concentrate on letting go of any residual tension. As you absorb the advantages of your practice, remain in Savasana for five to ten minutes.

4.4 Routine 4: Somatic Balance and Stability

Duration: 20 minutes

1. **Centering Breath**: Begin in a comfortable seated position with a tall spine. Close your eyes and take several deep breaths, focusing on filling your lungs completely with each inhale and emptying them fully with each exhale. Allow your breath to bring you into the present moment.

2. **Somatic Foot Activation**: Sit on the floor with legs extended. Point and flex your toes several times, then rotate your ankles in both directions. Spread your toes wide apart and then relax them. Repeat this foot activation sequence 5 times, focusing on increasing awareness and mobility in the feet.

3. **Somatic Hip Stability**: Lie on your back with knees bent and feet hip-width apart. Engage your core muscles and lift your hips off the ground into a bridge position. Hold for a few breaths, then slowly lower back down. Repeat this bridge pose 8-10 times, focusing on stability and control.

4. **Dynamic Balance Drill**: Stand with feet hip-width apart. Shift your weight onto your right foot and lift your left knee towards your chest, balancing on your right leg. Hold for a few breaths, then lower your left foot back down and repeat on the opposite side. Continue alternating between legs for 1 minute, focusing on maintaining balance and stability.

5. **Somatic Core Activation**: Sit on the floor with knees bent and feet flat on the ground. Place your hands behind your thighs and lean back slightly, engaging your core muscles. Hold this position for 10 seconds, then release and repeat 5 times, focusing on strengthening the abdominal muscles.

6. **Somatic Shoulder Stability**: Stand with feet hip-width apart and arms by your sides. Inhale as you reach your arms overhead, then exhale as you lower them back down, focusing on controlled movement and stability in the shoulders. Repeat this arm raise movement 8-10 times, synchronizing with your breath.

7. **Tree Pose:** Stand tall with feet hip-width apart. Shift your weight onto your right foot and place the sole of your left foot on the inside of your right thigh or calf, avoiding the knee joint. Put your hands together in the position of a prayer at your chest. After holding for a few breaths, switch sides. Repeat on each side for 3 rounds, focusing on finding balance and stability in the standing leg.

8. **Final Relaxation:** Lie down on your back in Savasana (Corpse Pose). Close your eyes and take several deep breaths, allowing your body to fully relax into the ground. Release any remaining tension from your muscles and surrender to a state of deep relaxation. Stay in Savasana for 5-10 minutes, enjoying the feeling of balance and stability within.

ADVANCED SOMATIC TECHNIQUES FOR PROGRESSION

In this section, we'll explore intermediate steps to further advance your somatic practice, building upon the foundational techniques learned in earlier chapters. These exercises are designed to deepen your body awareness, refine movement patterns, and enhance overall somatic proficiency.

1. Exploring Whole-Body Integration

Whole-body integration exercises focus on coordinating movements across multiple muscle groups and joints, promoting fluidity and efficiency in movement.

Standing Cat-Cow Stretch:
- Stand with your feet hip-width apart and arms by your sides.
- Inhale as you reach your arms overhead, arching your back slightly.
- Exhale as you round your spine, bringing your arms down towards your sides.

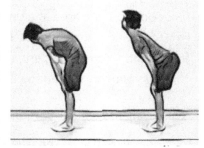

- Repeat this sequence for 10-15 repetitions, focusing on the integration of breath and movement.

Somatic Walking:
- Start off cautiously, focusing on how each body part moves.
- Observe how your weight shifts from one foot to the other and how your arms swing.
- Practice walking mindfully for 5-10 minutes, focusing on the sensations in your body with each step.

2. Deepening Body Awareness

Deepening body awareness exercises help you become more attuned to subtle sensations and movements within your body.

Body Scanning Meditation:
- Find a comfortable seated or lying position and close your eyes.
- Start at your feet and slowly scan your body from bottom to top, noticing any areas of tension or discomfort.
- Take deep breaths as you scan each body part, allowing any tension to release with each exhale.
- Continue scanning until you reach the top of your head, then take a few moments to observe the sensations in your entire body.

Somatic Sensory Exploration:
- Sit or lie down in a comfortable position and close your eyes.
- Begin to explore different sensations in your body, such as warmth, tingling, or heaviness.
- Focus on one area at a time, moving from your head down to your toes, and notice how each part of your body feels.
- Spend 5-10 minutes engaging in this sensory exploration, deepening your connection to your body's internal landscape.

3. Enhancing Movement Variability

Movement variability exercises encourage you to explore a wider range of motion and movement patterns, promoting adaptability and resilience in your body.

Spinal Articulation Sequence:
- Begin in a seated position with your legs extended in front of you.
- Slowly roll down through your spine, segment by segment, until your back is resting on the floor.
- Roll back up to a seated position, articulating through each vertebra.
- Repeat this sequence for 5-10 repetitions, focusing on smooth, controlled movements and maintaining awareness of your spine.

Dynamic Balance Challenges:
- Stand on one leg and slowly lift the opposite knee towards your chest.
- Hold the position for a few breaths, then extend the lifted leg straight out in front of you.
- Slowly return to the starting position and repeat on the opposite side.
- Perform 5-10 repetitions on each leg, focusing on maintaining balance and stability throughout the movement.

Incorporate these intermediate somatic practices into your routine to deepen your understanding of your body's movement patterns and enhance your overall somatic experience. Practice regularly and listen to your body's feedback to determine the appropriate level of challenge for your current skill level.

5.2 Breathwork Integration: Enhancing Somatic Awareness

In this section, we delve into the integration of breathwork techniques to deepen somatic awareness and enhance the mind-body connection. By incorporating specific breathing practices into your somatic exercises, you can amplify the benefits of your practice and cultivate a heightened sense of awareness and presence.

1. Diaphragmatic Breathing

Diaphragmatic breathing, also known as belly breathing, is a foundational breathwork technique that encourages deep, full breaths to promote relaxation and reduce stress.

Supine Diaphragmatic Breathing:
- Lie down on your back with your knees bent and feet flat on the floor.
- Place one hand on your abdomen and the other hand on your chest.
- Breathe deeply through your nose, letting your stomach expand as air enters your lungs.
- Exhale slowly through your mouth, feeling your abdomen gently fall.
- Repeat this cycle for several breaths, focusing on the expansion and contraction of your abdomen with each breath.

Seated Diaphragmatic Breathing:
- With your hands resting on your thighs and your feet flat on the floor, take a comfortable seat in a chair.
- As you take a deep breath through your nose and fill your lungs with air, your abdomen should expand.
- Exhale slowly through your mouth, allowing your abdomen to gently contract.
- Continue this rhythmic breathing pattern for several breaths, maintaining a relaxed and steady pace.

2. Coordinated Breath-Movement Sequences

Coordinating your breath with specific movements enhances somatic awareness and helps synchronize body and mind during exercise.

Inhale/Exhale Matching:
- Begin in a comfortable standing position with your arms by your sides.

- Inhale deeply as you raise your arms overhead, reaching towards the ceiling.
- Exhale slowly as you lower your arms back down to your sides.
- Breathe in as you expand and out as you contract to synchronize your movements with your breathing.
- Repeat this sequence for several repetitions, maintaining smooth and controlled movements.

3. Mindful Breathing Meditation

Mindful breathing meditation cultivates present moment awareness and deepens your connection to the breath as a focal point for attention.

Seated Mindful Breathing:
- Find a quiet and comfortable space to sit with your back straight and your hands resting on your lap.
- Close your eyes and bring your attention to the sensation of your breath entering and leaving your body.
- Notice the rise and fall of your abdomen with each inhalation and exhalation.
- Carefully return your attention to the breath, without passing judgment, if your thoughts stray.
- Continue this practice for several minutes, allowing yourself to fully immerse in the rhythm of your breath.

By integrating breathwork techniques into your somatic practice, you can deepen your awareness of the mind-body connection and enhance the therapeutic benefits of your exercises. Experiment with these techniques to discover what resonates best with your body and incorporate them into your daily routine for optimal well-being and vitality.

5.3 Partner and Group Exercises: Deepening Your Practice

In this section, we explore the dynamic realm of partner and group exercises, which offer unique opportunities for deepening your somatic practice through shared movement experiences. Partner and group exercises foster connection, communication, and collaboration while enhancing body awareness and interpersonal skills.

1. Partner Assisted Stretching

Partner assisted stretching involves one person providing gentle assistance to another person to deepen their stretch and increase flexibility.

Seated Hamstring Stretch:
- Sit on the floor with your legs extended in front of you.
- Your partner sits behind you and gently pushes on your back, encouraging you to fold forward from the hips.
- Hold the stretch for 20-30 seconds while breathing deeply.
- Switch roles and repeat the stretch with your partner.

2. Mirror Movement

Mirror movement exercises involve mirroring your partner's movements to enhance synchronization and coordination.

Standing Mirror Movement:
- Stand facing your partner with ample space between you.
- Begin to move slowly and fluidly, allowing your partner to mirror your movements.
- Explore different movements such as arm circles, side bends, and twists, maintaining eye contact and staying attuned to each other's rhythm.

3. Group Somatic Exploration:

Group somatic exploration involves collective movement experiences that encourage creativity, expression, and collaboration.

Circle of Trust:
- Form a circle with your group, standing shoulder to shoulder.
- Begin to sway gently from side to side, allowing the movement to ripple through the circle.
- As you sway, close your eyes and focus on the sensations in your body, tuning into the collective energy of the group.
- Gradually explore different movements such as reaching, stretching, and bending, allowing the group energy to guide your movements.

4. Partner Breathing Synchronization

Partner breathing exercises involve synchronizing your breath with your partner's breath to deepen relaxation and connection.

Seated Partner Breathing:
- Sit facing your partner, cross-legged on the floor.
- Place your hands on each other's shoulders or knees.
- Begin to breathe deeply and rhythmically, syncing your inhales and exhales with your partner's breath.
- Focus on the sensation of your breath merging with your partner's breath, creating a sense of unity and harmony.

5. Guided Partner Meditation

Guided partner meditation involves leading your partner through a meditation practice to promote relaxation and inner awareness.

Relaxation Meditation:
- Sit comfortably facing your partner, with your hands resting gently on each other's knees.
- Close your eyes and take several deep breaths together, allowing any tension to release with each exhale.
- Guide your partner through a relaxation meditation, directing their attention to different areas of the body and encouraging them to release any remaining tension.

- After the meditation, take a moment to share your experiences and reflections with each other.

6. Partner Resistance Training

Partner resistance training involves using your partner's resistance to build strength and stability in various muscle groups.

Leg Press with Partner Resistance:
- With your feet flat on the ground and your knees bent, lie on your back.
- Your partner stands at your feet and gently presses against the soles of your feet.
- Engage your leg muscles and push against your partner's resistance, straightening your legs.
- Hold for a few seconds, then slowly lower your legs back to the starting position.
- Repeat for several repetitions, alternating roles with your partner.

7. Group Balance Challenges

Group balance challenges encourage teamwork and coordination while improving balance and proprioception.

Circle Balance Challenge:
- Form a circle with your group, standing shoulder to shoulder.
- Each person lifts one foot off the ground and balances on the other foot.
- Gradually, begin to pass a small object, such as a ball or beanbag, around the circle while maintaining balance.
- Focus on staying centered and stable as you receive and pass the object, using your core muscles to support your balance.

8. Partner Relaxation Massage

Partner relaxation massage promotes relaxation and stress relief through gentle touch and massage techniques.

Back Massage with Partner:
- Sit back to back with your partner, cross-legged on the floor.
- Take turns giving and receiving a gentle back massage, using circular motions with your palms and fingers.
- Pay close attention to how much pressure is just right to release tension without hurting yourself.
- Communicate with your partner to ensure they are comfortable and adjust your technique as needed.
- Afterward, take a moment to express gratitude to your partner for the relaxation and support they provided.

By incorporating partner and group exercises into your somatic practice, you can enhance your experience, deepen your connection with others, and cultivate a sense of community and collaboration. Experiment with these exercises to discover new ways of moving, connecting, and supporting each other on your somatic journey.

5.4 Advanced Somatic Techniques for Progression: Dynamic Flow Routine

Duration: 30 minutes
1. **Warm-up (5 minutes)**
   - Begin in a comfortable standing position with feet hip-width apart.
   - Take slow, deep breaths, inhaling through the nose and exhaling through the mouth.
   - Perform gentle neck rolls, rolling the head slowly in one direction, then the other, for 30 seconds each.
   - Move into shoulder circles, lifting the shoulders up towards the ears, then rolling them back and down, for 30 seconds.
2. **Dynamic Somatic Movements (15 minutes)**
   - Start with spinal waves: Stand with feet hip-width apart, inhale and arch the back, exhale and round the spine, moving smoothly for 1 minute.

- Transition into pelvic tilts: Stand with hands on hips, inhale and tilt the pelvis forward, exhale and tilt it back, continuing for 1 minute.
- Proceed to hip circles: Stand with feet planted, hands on hips, and rotate the hips in a circular motion, alternating directions every 30 seconds.
- Move into leg swings: Stand tall, holding onto a stable surface for support, and swing one leg forward and backward, then switch sides, performing 15 swings on each leg.

3. **Strength and Stability (7 minutes)**
- Perform lunges: Step forward with one foot, bending both knees to lower the body towards the ground, then return to standing position. Repeat on the other side, alternating for 1 minute.
- Transition to squats: Stand with feet shoulder-width apart, lower the body into a squat position, then return to standing. Repeat for 1 minute.
- Engage in plank holds: Come into a plank position, with hands directly under shoulders and body in a straight line from head to heels. Hold for 30 seconds to 1 minute.

4. **Cool-down and Stretching (3 minutes)**
- Finish with gentle stretches: Perform a seated forward fold, reaching towards the toes and holding for 30 seconds.
- Follow with a seated twist, twisting the torso to one side and holding for 15 seconds, then repeating on the other side.
- Conclude with a brief relaxation in a comfortable seated or lying position, focusing on deep breaths and releasing tension.

SOMATIC EXERCISES
FOR EMOTIONAL WELL-BEING

6.1 Managing Stress and Anxiety through Somatic Movement

Through the practice of somatic movement, individuals can effectively manage and alleviate these symptoms, promoting a sense of calm and relaxation. In this section, we will explore various somatic techniques and exercises specifically designed to help individuals cope with stress and anxiety.

1. Diaphragmatic Breathing Technique

One of the most effective ways to reduce stress and anxiety is through diaphragmatic breathing, also known as belly breathing. This technique involves breathing deeply into the diaphragm, which triggers the body's relaxation response and helps calm the nervous system.

Instructions:
- Find a comfortable seated or lying position, placing one hand on your chest and the other on your abdomen.
- Breathe deeply through your nose, letting your belly swell up with the air in your lungs.
- Breathe out slowly through your mouth, letting your belly contract as you do so.
- Focus on the sensation of your breath moving in and out of your body, allowing any tension or stress to melt away with each exhale.
- Repeat this exercise for several minutes, gradually increasing the duration as you become more comfortable with the technique.

2. Progressive Muscle Relaxation (PMR)

Progressive muscle relaxation is a technique that involves systematically tensing and relaxing different muscle groups in the body to promote physical and mental relaxation. By deliberately tensing and then releasing muscle tension, individuals can learn to recognize and reduce muscular tension associated with stress and anxiety.

Instructions:
- Find a quiet and comfortable space where you can lie down or sit comfortably.
- Begin by tensing the muscles in your feet as tightly as you can, holding for a few seconds, and then releasing the tension completely.
- Move on to the muscles in your calves, thighs, buttocks, abdomen, chest, arms, shoulders, neck, and face, repeating the process of tensing and releasing each muscle group.
- As you tense each muscle group, focus on the sensation of tension building up and then melting away as you relax.
- Continue this process, working your way through the entire body, until you feel a deep sense of relaxation and calm.

3. Mindful Body Scan

A mindful body scan is a meditation practice that involves systematically bringing awareness to different parts of the body, noticing any sensations or areas of tension without judgment. By cultivating awareness of bodily sensations, individuals can learn to recognize and release areas of stress and tension, promoting relaxation and peace of mind.

Instructions:
- Find a comfortable lying or seated position, closing your eyes and bringing your attention to your breath.
- Begin to slowly scan through your body, starting at your toes and moving up through your feet, ankles, calves, knees, thighs, and so on, paying attention to any sensations you notice along the way.

- If you encounter areas of tension or discomfort, take a moment to breathe into that area, allowing it to soften and release with each exhale.
- Continue scanning through your body, bringing awareness to each part in turn, until you reach the crown of your head.
- Take a few moments to simply rest in this state of relaxed awareness, allowing yourself to fully experience the present moment without judgment or expectation.

Experiment with each exercise to discover which ones resonate most with you, and remember to practice regularly for optimal results.

6.2 Emotional Release Practices: Exploring Body-Mind Connection

Emotions are an integral part of the human experience, and they often manifest in physical sensations and bodily tensions. In this section, we will delve into various somatic practices aimed at facilitating emotional release by exploring the intricate connection between the body and mind. By engaging in these exercises, individuals can gain insight into their emotional patterns and find greater freedom and ease in their physical bodies.

1. Body Scan Meditation

The body scan meditation is a powerful practice for exploring the body-mind connection and promoting emotional release. By systematically bringing awareness to different parts of the body, individuals can uncover areas of tension or discomfort that may be linked to unresolved emotions.

Instructions:
- Find a comfortable seated or lying position, closing your eyes and bringing your attention to your breath.
- Begin to slowly scan through your body, starting at your feet and moving up through your legs, pelvis, abdomen, chest, arms, shoulders, neck, and head.

- Look over every body part, paying attention to any tense spots or sensations that emerge. Breathe into these areas for a moment, allowing each exhale to soften and release them.
- If you encounter any emotions or memories associated with specific body sensations, simply observe them without judgment or attachment, allowing them to arise and pass away on their own.
- Continue scanning through your body until you reach the crown of your head, bringing awareness to your entire body as a whole.

2. Grounding Exercises

Grounding exercises are designed to help individuals feel more connected to their bodies and the present moment, thereby promoting emotional stability and release. These exercises often involve bringing attention to the sensations of contact between the body and the ground, such as the feet on the floor or the sit bones in a chair.

Instructions:
- Find a comfortable standing or seated position, placing your feet firmly on the ground or floor.
- Take a few deep breaths, focusing on the sensation of your feet making contact with the ground. Picture yourself being anchored in the here and now by roots that grow deep into the ground from the soles of your feet.
- With each inhale, imagine drawing up energy and support from the earth into your body. With each exhale, imagine releasing any tension or negative emotions down into the earth to be transmuted and recycled.
- Continue this practice for several minutes, allowing yourself to feel grounded, centered, and supported by the earth beneath you.

3. Somatic Movement Exploration

Somatic movement exploration involves allowing the body to move freely and spontaneously, without judgment or expectation. By giving the body permission to express itself through movement, individuals can release pent-up emotions and find greater emotional clarity and balance.

Instructions:
- Find a comfortable space where you can move freely without restriction. Begin by standing or sitting with your eyes closed, allowing your body to sway and move in whatever way feels natural.
- Tune into the sensations and impulses arising within your body, allowing them to guide your movement. Notice any areas of tension or resistance, and gently explore them through gentle stretching or movement.
- As you move, allow any emotions or memories to surface and express themselves through your body. Trust in the wisdom of your body to release what is no longer serving you, allowing for greater emotional freedom and well-being.
- Continue this practice for as long as feels comfortable, allowing yourself to fully immerse in the experience of somatic movement exploration.

By incorporating these emotional release practices into your somatic practice, you can deepen your understanding of the body-mind connection and cultivate greater emotional resilience and well-being. Experiment with each exercise to discover which ones resonate most with you, and remember to approach them with openness, curiosity, and self-compassion.

6.3 Cultivating Emotional Balance: Strategies for Beginners

Emotional balance is essential for overall well-being, as it allows individuals to navigate life's ups and downs with greater resilience and equanimity. In this section, we will explore various strategies for cultivating emotional balance through somatic practices. These techniques are designed to help beginners develop greater awareness of their emotions and learn how to respond to them in a healthy and constructive manner.

1. Breath Awareness Meditation

Breath awareness meditation is a simple yet powerful practice for cultivating emotional balance. By bringing attention to the breath, individuals can learn to observe their emotions without becoming overwhelmed by them, fostering a sense of calm and inner peace.

Instructions:

- Find a comfortable seated position, closing your eyes and bringing your attention to your breath.
- Begin to observe the natural rhythm of your breath, noticing the sensations of air flowing in and out of your nostrils.
- As thoughts or emotions arise, simply acknowledge them without judgment, allowing them to come and go like passing clouds in the sky.
- Whenever you find your mind wandering, gently bring your focus back to your breath, using it as an anchor to the present moment.
- Continue this practice for several minutes, gradually extending the duration as you become more comfortable with it.

2. Body-Scan for Emotional Awareness

The body-scan technique is a valuable tool for developing emotional awareness by bringing attention to the physical sensations associated with different emotions. By tuning into the body's signals, individuals can gain insight into their emotional states and learn to respond to them in a healthy way.

3. Mindful Movement for Emotional Release

Mindful movement practices such as yoga or tai chi can be effective ways to release pent-up emotions and cultivate emotional balance. By moving the body with awareness and intention, individuals can channel their emotions in a positive and constructive direction.

Instructions:

- Choose a mindful movement practice that resonates with you, whether it's yoga, tai chi, or qigong.

- Begin with gentle warm-up exercises to prepare your body for movement, focusing on the sensations of stretching and opening.
- As you move through the practice, pay attention to the physical sensations and emotions that arise. Notice any areas of tension or resistance, and explore them with gentle movement and breath.
- Allow yourself to express any emotions that arise during the practice, whether it's through tears, laughter, or simply a sense of release.
- Finish the practice with a few moments of stillness and reflection, acknowledging the emotions you've experienced and cultivating gratitude for the opportunity to move and breathe.

4. Mindful Journaling for Emotional Processing

Mindful journaling is a powerful tool for processing and understanding emotions, allowing individuals to explore their thoughts and feelings in a safe and non-judgmental space. By putting pen to paper, individuals can gain clarity and insight into their emotional experiences, fostering greater self-awareness and emotional resilience.

Instructions:
- Set aside time each day to engage in mindful journaling, choosing a quiet and comfortable space where you can focus without distractions.
- Begin by reflecting on your emotional experiences from the day, noting any significant events or interactions that elicited strong feelings.
- Let your ideas and feelings flow onto the page as you write freely and without fear of criticism. Avoid censoring or editing yourself; instead, let your words flow naturally.
- As you write, pay attention to the physical sensations in your body, noticing any areas of tension or discomfort. Use these sensations as cues to explore deeper into your emotions.

- After you've finished writing, take a few moments to review what you've written, noticing any patterns or insights that emerge. Consider how you can apply these insights to cultivate greater emotional balance in your life.

5. Self-Compassion Practices for Emotional Resilience

Self-compassion is an essential component of emotional resilience, allowing individuals to respond to their own suffering with kindness and understanding. By cultivating self-compassion, individuals can build a strong foundation for emotional well-being and develop greater resilience in the face of life's challenges.

Instructions:
- Begin by bringing awareness to any self-critical thoughts or beliefs that arise in your mind. Notice how these thoughts make you feel and how they impact your emotional state.
- Challenge the validity of these self-critical thoughts by asking yourself if they are based on reality or if they are simply habitual patterns of thinking. Remind yourself that everyone experiences difficulties and setbacks, and that you are not alone in your struggles.
- Give yourself encouraging and kind words as a way to practice self-compassion. Treat yourself with the same warmth and compassion that you would offer to a close friend or loved one.
- Engage in self-care activities that nourish your body, mind, and spirit, such as taking a warm bath, going for a walk in nature, or spending time with loved ones.
- Keep in mind that developing self-compassion is a skill that takes practice. Be patient with yourself and continue to nurture self-compassion as a cornerstone of your emotional resilience.

6. Gratitude Practices for Cultivating Emotional Balance

Gratitude is a powerful antidote to negative emotions, allowing individuals to shift their focus from what is lacking to what is abundant in their lives. By cultivating gratitude, individuals can foster a sense of appreciation and contentment, even in the face of adversity.

Instructions:

- Begin each day by taking a few moments to reflect on what you are grateful for in your life. Consider the people, experiences, and blessings that bring you joy and fulfillment.
- Keep a gratitude journal where you can regularly write down three things you are grateful for each day. This practice can help train your brain to focus on the positive aspects of your life, rather than dwelling on the negative.
- Practice expressing gratitude to others by writing thank-you notes or simply telling them how much you appreciate their presence in your life. Cultivate an attitude of gratitude in your interactions with others, and notice how it impacts your relationships and overall sense of well-being.
- When faced with challenges or difficulties, try to find something to be grateful for, even if it's small. This shift in perspective can help you approach problems with greater resilience and creativity.

SOMATIC EXERCISES FOR PAIN MANAGEMENT

Pain relief through somatic techniques is a transformative journey that empowers individuals to reclaim control over their bodies and alleviate discomfort naturally. By understanding the underlying principles and practicing specific somatic exercises, individuals can cultivate a profound awareness of their bodies and unlock the potential for lasting pain relief.

Introduction to Somatic Pain Relief

Somatic pain relief involves a holistic approach to understanding and addressing the root causes of physical discomfort. Unlike traditional methods that focus solely on symptom management, somatic techniques delve deeper into the body-mind connection to uncover and release muscular tension, improve posture, and restore balance.

Principles of Somatic Pain Relief

Central to somatic pain relief is the principle of sensory-motor awareness, which emphasizes the importance of consciously sensing and moving muscles to alleviate tension and pain. By cultivating awareness of habitual movement patterns and releasing chronic muscular contractions, individuals can experience profound relief from pain and discomfort.

Exploring Muscle Release Patterns

Muscle release patterns are specific sequences of movements designed to target and release tension in key areas of the body. By systematically engaging and relaxing muscles, individuals can interrupt the cycle of chronic muscular contraction and promote relaxation and pain relief.

Exercise: Shoulder Melting

- Start by taking a comfortable seat or standing with your shoulders relaxed and your spine straight.
- Inhale deeply, and as you exhale, gently lift your shoulders towards your ears, feeling the tension in your upper trapezius muscles.
- Hold this tension for a few seconds, then slowly and deliberately release the shoulders downwards, allowing them to "melt" away from your ears.
- Repeat this movement several times, focusing on the sensation of tension release with each repetition. Notice any changes in the sensation of your shoulders and neck as you continue the exercise.

Breathwork for Pain Management

Breathwork is a powerful tool for managing pain and promoting relaxation throughout the body. By incorporating conscious breathing techniques into somatic practice, individuals can reduce muscular tension, calm the nervous system, and enhance overall well-being.

Exercise: Diaphragmatic Breathing

Practice the technique as explained in the previous chapters.

Integrating Somatic Practices into Daily Life

The key to long-term pain relief is the integration of somatic practices into daily life. By incorporating mindful movement, breathwork, and relaxation techniques into everyday activities, individuals can cultivate greater body awareness and resilience to stressors.

Practice: Somatic Walking

- Bring attention to your feet as you walk, noticing the sensation of each step connecting with the ground.
- Pay attention to the alignment of your body, keeping your spine tall and your shoulders relaxed.
- Take slow, deliberate steps, focusing on the quality of movement rather than speed. Notice how your body responds to each movement and adjust accordingly to promote ease and comfort.
- As you walk, incorporate diaphragmatic breathing and gentle movements to enhance relaxation and promote a sense of well-being.

7.2 Techniques for Alleviating Headaches and Tension

Headaches and tension are common ailments that can significantly impact daily life. Fortunately, somatic techniques offer practical solutions for alleviating these symptoms and promoting overall well-being. By integrating mindful movement, breathwork, and relaxation techniques, individuals can effectively manage headaches and tension, restoring balance and harmony to the body.

Understanding Headaches and Tension

Headaches and tension often result from muscular contractions and imbalances in the neck, shoulders, and upper back. These areas are particularly prone to stress and strain due to poor posture, repetitive movements, and emotional stressors. By addressing the underlying muscular tension and promoting relaxation, individuals can experience relief from headaches and tension.

Breathwork for Headache Relief

Breathwork is a powerful tool for alleviating headaches and tension, as it helps to calm the nervous system, reduce stress, and promote relaxation throughout the body. By incorporating specific breathing techniques into somatic practice, individuals can effectively manage headaches and prevent their recurrence.

Exercise: Three-Part Breath
- Find a comfortable seated or lying position, with your spine tall and your shoulders relaxed.
- Place one hand on your abdomen and the other hand on your chest.
- Inhale deeply through your nose, allowing your abdomen to expand fully as you fill your lungs with air. Feel your chest rise slightly.
- Feel the contraction and deflation of your abdomen as you slowly and fully exhale through your mouth. Notice the sensation of relaxation spreading throughout your body with each exhalation.
- For several minutes, keep repeating these three-part breaths, allowing each one to take you farther into a deeper state of relaxation.

Neck and Shoulder Release Techniques

Targeted exercises for the neck and shoulders can help to release tension and alleviate headaches. By gently mobilizing the neck and shoulders, individuals can improve circulation, reduce muscular tightness, and promote relaxation in these areas.

Exercise: Neck Rolls
- Sit or stand in a comfortable position with your spine tall and your shoulders relaxed.
- Inhale deeply and as you exhale, slowly lower your chin towards your chest, feeling a gentle stretch along the back of your neck.
- Inhale again and as you exhale, slowly roll your head to the right, bringing your right ear towards your right shoulder. Pause for a moment and then inhale as you return to center.
- Repeat the movement to the left side, bringing your left ear towards your left shoulder. Continue to alternate sides, moving with the rhythm of your breath.

Self-Massage Techniques

Self-massage techniques can also be effective for relieving headaches and tension by releasing muscular knots and promoting circulation. By applying gentle pressure to specific trigger points, individuals can alleviate discomfort and promote relaxation in the affected areas.

Exercise: Scalp Massage
- Sit or stand comfortably with your spine tall and your shoulders relaxed.
- Using your fingertips, begin massaging your scalp in circular motions, starting at the base of your skull and moving towards the crown of your head.
- Apply gentle pressure as you massage, paying attention to any areas of tension or discomfort. Continue massaging for several minutes, focusing on promoting relaxation and relieving muscular tightness.

7.3 Managing Joint Discomfort with Somatic Practices

Joint discomfort can significantly impact daily activities and quality of life, but somatic practices offer effective techniques for managing and alleviating this discomfort. By focusing on gentle movements, breathwork, and mindfulness, individuals can enhance joint mobility, reduce stiffness, and promote overall joint health. This comprehensive approach targets the root causes of joint discomfort, empowering individuals to take control of their well-being and live with greater ease and comfort.

Understanding Joint Discomfort

Joint discomfort can arise from various factors, including injury, overuse, inflammation, and age-related changes. Common areas affected include the knees, hips, shoulders, and wrists. Symptoms may range from mild stiffness and achiness to sharp or shooting pains during movement. By understanding the underlying causes of joint discomfort, individuals can tailor their somatic practice to address specific areas of concern and promote optimal joint function.

Breathwork for Joint Mobility

Breathwork plays a crucial role in somatic practices for managing joint discomfort. By cultivating awareness of the breath and incorporating specific breathing techniques, individuals can reduce tension, improve circulation, and enhance relaxation throughout the body. Deep, diaphragmatic breathing encourages the release of tension in the muscles surrounding the joints, promoting greater mobility and comfort.

Exercise: Diaphragmatic Breathing
- Find a comfortable seated or lying position, with your spine tall and your shoulders relaxed.
- Place one hand on your abdomen and the other hand on your chest.
- Inhale deeply through your nose, allowing your abdomen to expand fully as you fill your lungs with air. Feel your hand rise with the expansion of your belly.
- Feel the contraction and deflation of your abdomen as you slowly and fully exhale through your mouth. Notice the sensation of relaxation spreading throughout your body with each exhalation.
- Repeat this diaphragmatic breathing for several minutes, allowing yourself to relax more deeply with each breath.

Gentle Joint Mobilization Exercises

Gentle joint mobilization exercises can help to reduce stiffness and increase range of motion, promoting comfort and ease in daily movements. These exercises focus on slow, controlled movements that gently stretch and mobilize the joints, helping to lubricate them and improve their function over time.

Exercise: Wrist Circles
- Extend your arms in front of you at shoulder height, palms facing down.

- Begin making slow circles with your wrists, moving in a clockwise direction. Focus on moving from the wrists while keeping the rest of your arms and shoulders relaxed.
- After several circles, reverse direction and make circles in a counterclockwise direction.
- Continue this movement for several repetitions, breathing deeply and maintaining a sense of ease and relaxation.

Mindful Movement for Joint Health

Mindful movement practices, such as tai chi and qigong, can also be beneficial for managing joint discomfort. These practices emphasize slow, deliberate movements that promote balance, coordination, and flexibility. By incorporating mindful movement into their somatic practice, individuals can improve joint health and reduce discomfort while cultivating a sense of peace and tranquility.

Exercise: Tai Chi-Inspired Arm Swings
- Stand with your feet shoulder-width apart, knees slightly bent, and spine tall.
- Begin swinging your arms gently from side to side, allowing them to float freely with the movement of your body.
- Coordinate your breath with your movements, inhaling as your arms swing forward and exhaling as they swing backward.
- Continue this fluid motion for several minutes, allowing yourself to relax and soften with each swing.

INTEGRATING SOMATIC MOVEMENT INTO DAILY LIFE

8.1 Incorporating Somatic Practices into Everyday Activities

Integrating somatic practices into daily life offers a profound opportunity to cultivate mindfulness, enhance body awareness, and promote overall well-being. By infusing simple somatic techniques into familiar routines and activities, individuals can experience greater ease, comfort, and vitality throughout their day. From sitting at a desk to walking in nature, there are countless opportunities to engage with somatic principles and reap the benefits of embodied living.

Mindful Movement in Daily Tasks

Mindful movement involves bringing focused attention and awareness to the body's movements and sensations during everyday activities. By practicing mindfulness while performing tasks such as walking, standing, or reaching, individuals can enhance proprioception, reduce tension, and improve posture and alignment.

Exercise: Mindful Walking
- Begin by standing tall with your feet hip-width apart and your arms relaxed by your sides.
- To center yourself and focus on the here and now, take a few deep breaths.
- Slowly begin to walk, paying close attention to the sensation of each step as your foot makes contact with the ground.

- Notice the subtle shifts in weight and balance with each movement, allowing yourself to move with ease and grace.
- If your thoughts stray, gently return them to the sensation of walking and the cadence of your breathing.
- Continue walking mindfully for several minutes, allowing yourself to fully immerse in the experience.

Somatic Awareness in Sitting

Many people spend prolonged periods sitting throughout the day, whether at work, during meals, or while commuting. Incorporating somatic awareness into sitting activities can help prevent discomfort and promote healthy alignment.

Exercise: Somatic Sitting
- Find a comfortable chair with a firm, supportive seat and a straight back.
- Sit with your feet flat on the floor and your spine tall, allowing your shoulders to relax down away from your ears.
- Close your eyes and take a few deep breaths to center yourself and bring awareness to your body.
- Begin to notice the points of contact between your body and the chair, feeling the sensation of support beneath you.
- Scan your body for areas of tension or discomfort, and gently release any tension as you continue to breathe deeply.
- Maintain this somatic awareness while sitting, periodically checking in with your body and making any necessary adjustments to promote comfort and alignment.

Breathwork for Stress Relief

Breathwork is a powerful tool for managing stress and promoting relaxation throughout the day. By incorporating simple breathing exercises into daily activities, individuals can calm the nervous system, reduce tension, and enhance overall well-being.

Exercise: Calming Breath
- Find a quiet space where you can sit or stand comfortably.
- Close your eyes and take a few deep breaths to settle into the present moment.
- Inhale deeply through your nose for a count of four, allowing your abdomen to expand fully with each breath.
- Exhale slowly and completely through your mouth for a count of six, releasing any tension or stress with each breath.
- Continue this rhythmic breathing pattern for several minutes, allowing yourself to relax more deeply with each exhalation.

8.2 Workplace Wellness: Somatic Strategies for Stress Reduction

In today's fast-paced work environments, stress has become a common companion for many individuals. However, incorporating somatic strategies into the workplace can offer effective tools for managing stress, enhancing well-being, and promoting productivity. By integrating simple somatic practices into the workday, employees can cultivate greater resilience, focus, and overall job satisfaction.

Mindful Movement Breaks

Taking short breaks throughout the workday to engage in mindful movement can help alleviate stress and tension, improve circulation, and boost energy levels. These brief pauses provide an opportunity to reconnect with the body, release muscular tension, and recharge mental focus.

Exercise: Desk Stretching
- Begin by sitting tall in your chair with your feet flat on the floor and your hands resting gently on your thighs.
- Inhale deeply as you reach both arms overhead, lengthening through the spine and fingertips.
- Exhale slowly as you gently lean to one side, stretching through the side body.

- Hold the stretch for a few breaths, feeling the lengthening sensation along the opposite side of your torso.
- Inhale to return to center, then exhale as you repeat the stretch on the opposite side.
- Continue to alternate sides for several repetitions, moving with the rhythm of your breath.

Breathwork for Stress Relief

Conscious breathing techniques can be powerful allies in the battle against workplace stress. By practicing simple breathwork exercises, employees can activate the body's relaxation response, calm the mind, and regain a sense of balance and clarity.

Exercise: Box Breathing
- Find a comfortable seated position with your feet flat on the floor and your hands resting lightly on your lap.
- Close your eyes and take a few deep breaths to settle into the present moment.
- Inhale slowly and deeply through your nose for a count of four, feeling your abdomen expand with each breath.
- Hold the breath for a count of four at the top of the inhale, maintaining a sense of fullness and presence.
- Exhale slowly and completely through your mouth for a count of four, allowing any tension or stress to melt away.
- Hold the breath out for a count of four before beginning the next inhalation.
- Repeat this box breathing pattern for several cycles, allowing yourself to relax more deeply with each breath.

Mindful Eating Practices

Incorporating mindfulness into meals and snack breaks can transform eating from a mindless habit into a nourishing self-care practice. By savoring each bite, paying attention to hunger and fullness cues, and cultivating gratitude for the nourishment received, employees can enhance digestion, reduce stress-related eating, and foster a healthier relationship with food.

Exercise: Mindful Eating Meditation
- Begin by selecting a small snack or meal to enjoy mindfully, such as a piece of fruit or a cup of tea.
- Find a quiet space where you can sit comfortably without distractions.
- To center yourself and focus on the here and now, take a few deep breaths.
- Notice the colors, textures, and aromas of your food, allowing yourself to fully appreciate its sensory qualities.
- Take a small bite or sip, and pay close attention to the taste, texture, and temperature of the food.
- Chew slowly and mindfully, savoring each bite and allowing yourself to fully experience the flavors.
- Observe, without bias or attachment, any thoughts or feelings that surface during your meal.
- Continue to eat in this mindful manner until you feel satisfied and nourished.

Whether through mindful movement breaks, breathwork exercises, or mindful eating practices, there are countless opportunities to reduce stress and promote wellness throughout the workday.

8.3 Promoting Better Sleep and Relaxation with Somatics

In today's fast-paced world, many individuals struggle with sleep disturbances and difficulty relaxing due to the demands of modern life. However, integrating somatic practices into your bedtime routine can be a powerful tool for promoting better sleep and deep relaxation. By engaging in gentle movements, breathwork, and mindfulness techniques, you can create a conducive environment for restful sleep and rejuvenation.

Creating a Relaxing Bedtime Ritual

Establishing a soothing bedtime ritual can signal to your body and mind that it's time to unwind and prepare for sleep. By incorporating somatic practices into your nightly routine, you can release tension, quiet the mind, and set the stage for a restful night's sleep.

Exercise: Evening Body Scan

- Begin by lying comfortably in bed with your eyes closed and your body fully supported by the mattress.
- Take a few deep breaths to center yourself and bring your awareness into the present moment.
- Starting from your toes, gradually scan your body from head to toe, noticing any areas of tension or discomfort.
- As you identify areas of tension, consciously release the muscles and invite a sense of relaxation to wash over you.
- Continue this body scan technique, moving slowly and mindfully through each area of your body, until you reach the crown of your head.
- Take a few moments to bask in the sensation of relaxation that permeates your entire body, allowing yourself to fully surrender to the present moment.

Breathwork for Relaxation

Utilizing specific breathwork techniques can help calm the nervous system, quiet the mind, and promote a state of deep relaxation conducive to sleep. By harnessing the power of the breath, you can release tension, reduce stress, and facilitate the transition into restful slumber.

Exercise: 4-7-8 Breathing

- Find a comfortable lying position in bed, with your arms resting gently by your sides and your eyes closed.
- Inhale deeply through your nose for a count of four, allowing your abdomen to rise and fill with air.
- Hold your breath at the top of the inhale for a count of seven, feeling a sense of fullness and expansion in your chest.

- Exhale slowly and completely through your mouth for a count of eight, allowing any remaining tension or stress to melt away.
- Repeat this 4-7-8 breathing pattern for several rounds, allowing each breath to deepen your sense of relaxation and peace.

Gentle Movement for Release

Incorporating gentle somatic movements into your bedtime routine can help release accumulated tension, promote circulation, and prepare your body for restorative sleep. These simple movements can be performed directly in bed, allowing you to seamlessly transition from wakefulness to sleep.

Exercise: Supine Twist
- Begin by lying on your back in bed with your arms extended out to the sides, palms facing down.
- Bend your knees and draw them in toward your chest, keeping your feet flat on the bed.
- Exhale as you gently lower both knees to one side, allowing them to come to rest on the bed.
- Keep your shoulders grounded as you turn your head in the opposite direction, feeling a gentle stretch through your spine and lower back.
- Hold the twist for several breaths, allowing your body to soften and release with each exhale.
- Inhale to return to center, then exhale as you repeat the twist on the opposite side.
- Continue to move slowly and mindfully through each repetition, allowing your body to relax more deeply with each twist.

WEIGHT LOSS PROGRAM
WITH SOMATIC EXERCISES

9.1 Introduction to Weight Loss with Somatics

In our journey towards achieving and maintaining a healthy weight, somatic practices offer a unique and effective approach that goes beyond traditional diet and exercise routines. By cultivating awareness of our body's sensations and movement patterns, we can develop a deeper understanding of the underlying causes of weight gain and implement sustainable strategies for long-term success. In this section, we will explore the principles of somatics as they relate to weight loss and introduce practical techniques for incorporating somatic practices into your daily routine.

Understanding the Mind-Body Connection

Central to the somatic approach to weight loss is the recognition of the intricate connection between the mind and body. Our thoughts, emotions, and beliefs about food, exercise, and body image can significantly influence our behaviors and habits related to weight management. By cultivating awareness of these internal factors, we can begin to unravel unhealthy patterns and develop a more balanced and mindful approach to eating and movement.

Exercise: Body Scan Meditation

Cultivating Mindful Eating Habits

Incorporating mindfulness into our eating habits can profoundly impact our relationship with food and support our weight loss goals. By paying attention to the sensory experience of eating, we can become more attuned to hunger and satiety cues, make healthier food choices, and prevent overeating.

Exercise: Mindful Eating Practice
- Before each meal or snack, take a few moments to pause and center yourself.
- Notice the appearance, aroma, and texture of the food in front of you, engaging all of your senses.
- Take a small bite of food and chew slowly, savoring the flavors and textures as they unfold in your mouth.
- Pay attention to the sensations of hunger and fullness, as well as any emotional triggers that arise during the eating process.
- Avoid distractions such as television or electronic devices, allowing yourself to fully focus on the experience of eating.
- Practice gratitude for the nourishment and pleasure that food provides, fostering a positive and balanced relationship with eating.

Movement as Medicine

Physical activity is an essential component of any weight loss program, but traditional exercise routines can sometimes feel daunting or unsustainable. Somatic movement practices offer a gentle and intuitive approach to movement that focuses on improving body awareness, flexibility, and strength while reducing tension and stress.

Exercise: Somatic Movement Sequence
- Begin in a comfortable standing position with your feet hip-width apart and your arms relaxed by your sides.
- Take a few deep breaths to center yourself and connect with your body.

- Slowly begin to sway from side to side, allowing your arms to swing freely and your spine to gently mobilize.
- Gradually increase the range of motion as you sway, exploring the full range of movement available to you.
- Notice any areas of stiffness or restriction in your body and invite gentle movement and relaxation into those areas.
- Continue swaying for several minutes, allowing the rhythm of your breath to guide your movements.
- As you conclude the practice, take a moment to notice how your body feels and express gratitude for the opportunity to move and connect with yourself.

9.2 Warm-up Routine for Weight Loss

As we embark on our journey towards weight loss, it's essential to prepare our bodies for movement with a thorough warm-up routine. A proper warm-up not only helps prevent injury but also primes our muscles and joints for the physical activity ahead. In this section, we will explore a comprehensive warm-up routine specifically designed to support weight loss goals. Each exercise is carefully selected to engage multiple muscle groups, increase flexibility, and elevate heart rate, setting the stage for a successful workout session.

1. Dynamic Stretching

Controlled motions that gradually extend your muscles and joints through their entire range of motion are the basis of dynamic stretching. Stretching like this is especially good for increasing flexibility and body temperature.

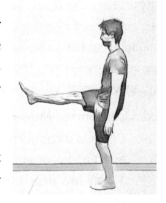

Exercise: Leg Swings
- Stand tall with your feet hip-width apart and hold onto a sturdy support for balance.

- Swing one leg forward and backward in a controlled motion, keeping your torso upright and your core engaged.
- Gradually increase the range of motion with each swing, aiming to lift your leg higher with each repetition.
- Perform 10-15 swings on each leg, focusing on maintaining smooth and fluid movement.

2. Cardiovascular Activation

Elevating your heart rate is crucial for preparing your body for aerobic exercise and optimizing calorie burn during your workout. Cardiovascular activation exercises help increase blood flow to your muscles and enhance overall circulation.

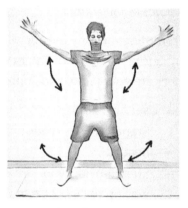

Exercise: Jumping Jacks
- Start with your feet together and your arms by your sides.
- At the same time as you raise your arms overhead, jump with your feet spread wide.
- Return to the starting position by jumping your feet back together and lowering your arms to your sides.
- Continue performing jumping jacks for 1-2 minutes, maintaining a steady pace and focusing on controlled movements.

3. Core Activation

A strong core is essential for maintaining proper posture, stability, and balance during exercise. Core activation exercises help engage the muscles of your abdomen, lower back, and pelvis, setting a solid foundation for effective workouts.

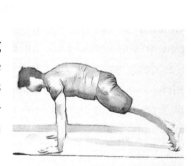

Exercise: Plank
- Begin in a push-up position with your hands directly beneath your shoulders and your body forming a straight line from head to heels.
- Engage your core muscles and hold this position for 30-60 seconds, focusing on keeping your spine neutral and your hips level.
- Avoid sagging or arching your back, and breathe deeply throughout the exercise to maintain stability.

4. Joint Mobilization

Promoting mobility in your joints is essential for preventing stiffness and enhancing overall movement efficiency. Joint mobilization exercises help lubricate your joints and improve their range of motion.

Exercise: Arm Circles
- Stand tall with your arms extended out to your sides at shoulder height.
- Start moving your arms in small, circular motions and work your way up to larger circles.
- Continue circling your arms for 1-2 minutes, alternating between clockwise and counterclockwise rotations.

9.3 Core Strengthening Exercises for Weight Loss

When it comes to achieving weight loss goals, building a strong core is paramount. Not only does a strong core improve posture and stability, but it also enhances overall functional movement and helps support the spine. In this section, we will explore a series of core strengthening exercises designed to target the muscles of the abdomen, lower back, and pelvis. These exercises are beginner-friendly and can be performed virtually anywhere, making them ideal for incorporating into your weight loss routine.

1. Plank Variations

The plank is a fundamental core exercise that targets multiple muscle groups simultaneously, including the abdominals, obliques, and lower back. By holding a plank position, you engage your core muscles isometrically, helping to build strength and stability.

Exercise: Forearm Plank

- Begin by lying face down on the floor with your elbows bent and directly beneath your shoulders.
- Lift your body off the ground, supporting your weight on your forearms and toes.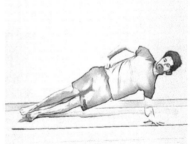
- Engage your core muscles to maintain a straight line from your head to your heels, avoiding any sagging or arching of the back.
- Hold this position for 30-60 seconds, focusing on steady breathing and maintaining proper form.

Exercise: Side Plank

- Start by lying on your side with your legs extended and your elbow positioned directly beneath your shoulder.
- Raise your hips off the floor so that your head and heels are in a straight line.
- Engage your core muscles and hold this position for 30-60 seconds on each side, keeping your body stable and aligned.

2. Bicycle Crunches

Bicycle crunches are an effective exercise for targeting the rectus abdominis and oblique muscles, helping to sculpt and define your midsection.

Exercise: Bicycle Crunches

- Lie on your back with your knees bent and your hands placed lightly behind your head.
- Raise your shoulders off the floor and extend your right elbow to your left knee while extending your right leg straight ahead.

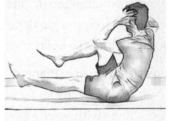

- Rotate your torso and bring your left elbow towards your right knee as you extend your left leg.
- Continue alternating sides in a pedaling motion, focusing on engaging your core muscles with each repetition.

3. Russian Twists

Russian twists are a dynamic core exercise that targets the obliques and improves rotational strength.

Exercise: Russian Twists

- Sit on the floor with your knees bent and your feet flat on the ground.
- Using your sit bones for balance, slant your back a little and raise your feet off the ground.
- Clasp your hands together in front of your chest and rotate your torso to the right, bringing your hands towards the floor beside your hip.

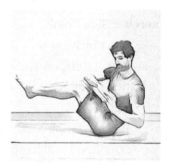

- Return to the center and then rotate to the left, bringing your hands towards the floor on the opposite side.
- Continue alternating sides in a controlled manner, focusing on maintaining balance and stability.

Certainly! Let's continue exploring core strengthening exercises for weight loss:

4. Dead Bug

The dead bug exercise is a fantastic way to target the deep core muscles while also improving coordination and stability.

Exercise: Dead Bug

- Begin by lying on your back with your arms extended towards the ceiling and your legs bent at a 90-degree angle, knees stacked over hips.
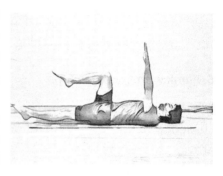
- Engage your core muscles to press your lower back into the floor, maintaining a neutral spine.
- Slowly lower your right arm overhead towards the floor while simultaneously straightening your left leg, hovering it just above the ground.
- Step back to the beginning and repeat on the other side, alternating sides under control.
- Focus on keeping your core engaged throughout the movement to stabilize the spine and pelvis.

5. Bird Dog

The bird dog exercise is another effective way to strengthen the core muscles while also improving balance and coordination.

Exercise: Bird Dog

- Begin on your hands and knees in a tabletop position, with your wrists aligned under your shoulders and your knees under your hips.
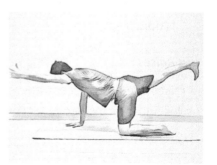
- Engage your core muscles to stabilize your spine, keeping

your back flat and neck neutral.

- Extend your right arm forward and your left leg back, maintaining a straight line from your fingertips to your heel.
- Hold this position briefly, then return to the starting position and switch sides, extending your left arm and right leg.
- Focus on maintaining balance and stability throughout the movement, avoiding any arching or rounding of the back.

6. Plank with Shoulder Taps

Adding a dynamic element to the traditional plank exercise increases the challenge to the core muscles while also engaging the shoulders and arms.

Exercise: Plank with Shoulder Taps

- Begin in a forearm plank position, with your elbows bent and directly beneath your shoulders, and your body in a straight line from head to heels.

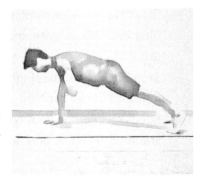

- Engage your core muscles to keep your hips stable as you lift your right hand off the ground and tap your left shoulder.
- Return to the starting position and repeat on the opposite side, tapping your right shoulder with your left hand.
- Continue alternating sides while maintaining a strong plank position, focusing on keeping your hips square and minimizing any rotation.

7. Leg Raises

Leg raises are an excellent exercise for targeting the lower abdominal muscles and improving overall core strength.

Exercise: Leg Raises

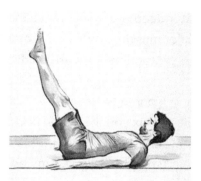

- Lie on your back with your legs extended and your arms resting by your sides, palms facing down.
- Engage your core muscles to press your lower back into the floor, keeping your spine neutral.
- When your legs are perpendicular to the floor, slowly raise them off the ground while keeping them straight and together.
- Lower your legs back down towards the ground with control, stopping just before they touch the floor, and then lift them back up.
- Focus on using your abdominal muscles to lift and lower your legs, avoiding any swinging or momentum.

9.4 Cool-down and Stretching for Weight Loss

As you wrap up your weight loss workout, it's crucial to transition your body from high-intensity exercise to a state of relaxation and recovery. Incorporating a thorough cool-down and stretching routine not only helps prevent muscle soreness and injury but also promotes flexibility and mobility, supporting your overall fitness journey.

1. Deep Breathing

Begin your cool-down with a few minutes of deep breathing to help lower your heart rate and promote relaxation. Take a seat or lie down where you feel comfortable, close your eyes, and inhale deeply through your nose and exhale slowly through your mouth. Focus on filling your lungs with air and releasing any tension or stress with each exhale.

2. Full-Body Stretch

After deep breathing, move into a full-body stretching routine to target major muscle groups and promote flexibility.

- **Standing Forward Fold**: Stand with your feet hip-width apart and slowly hinge forward at the hips, allowing your torso to fold over your legs. Reach towards the ground or grab opposite elbows and relax your head and neck.
- **Chest Opener**: Interlace your fingers behind your back and straighten your arms as you lift your chest towards the ceiling, opening up through the front of your body.
- **Seated Spinal Twist**: Sit on the ground with your legs extended in front of you. With your right foot level on the ground, bend your right knee and cross it over your left leg. Your left elbow should be on the outside of your right knee when you turn your torso to the right and glance over your right shoulder. Repeat on the other side.
- **Child's Pose**: Kneel on the ground with your big toes touching and knees spread apart. With your forehead resting on the floor, extend your arms forward while sitting back on your heels. Relax your entire body and focus on deepening your breath.

3. Targeted Muscle Stretches

Following a full-body stretch, focus on stretching specific muscle groups that may have been particularly engaged during your workout.

- **Hamstring Stretch**: Lie on your back with one leg extended on the ground and the other leg lifted towards the ceiling. Hold onto the back of your thigh or calf and gently pull your leg towards your chest, feeling a stretch in the back of your thigh. Repeat on the other side.
- **Quadriceps Stretch**: Taking a strong stance, reach back and bring one foot to your glutes. Feel a stretch in the front of your thigh and maintain your body upright while keeping your knees close together. For balance, cling to a chair or wall if necessary.
- **Calf Stretch**: Place one foot in front of you and one behind you as you face a wall. Bend your front knee and keep your rear leg

straight as you lean forward and press your hands against the wall. Your calf muscle ought to feel stretched. Continue on the opposite side.

4. Relaxation Techniques

Finish your cool-down with relaxation techniques to promote mental and physical recovery.

- **Body Scan Meditation:**Closing your eyes, lie on your back. Bring your awareness to each part of your body, starting from your toes and gradually moving up to your head. With every exhalation, identify any tight spots or uncomfortable spots and deliberately release them.
- **Visualization:** Visualize yourself achieving your weight loss goals and feeling strong, healthy, and vibrant. Imagine yourself moving through your workouts with ease and confidence, embodying the changes you wish to see in your body and life.

STRESS RELIEF PROGRAM FOR BEGINNERS

10.1 Comprehending the Impact of Stress on the Human Body

Stress is an intricate interplay between our minds and bodies, a natural response ingrained in our biology to help us navigate life's challenges. At its core, stress is our body's way of mobilizing resources to deal with perceived threats or demands, whether they be physical, emotional, or psychological.

Stress sets forth a series of physiological reactions that prime us for action. When we encounter a stressful situation, our sympathetic nervous system kicks into gear, releasing hormones like adrenaline and cortisol into the bloodstream. These hormones prime us to either fight or run from the perceived threat by raising blood pressure, speeding up the pulse rate, and rerouting blood supply to vital organs.

However, chronic or prolonged stress can take a toll on our bodies. Persistent muscle tension, particularly in areas like the neck, shoulders, and back, can lead to discomfort and pain. Digestive issues, such as stomach cramps or indigestion, may arise as stress disrupts normal digestive processes. Sleep disturbances are common, as stress hormones interfere with our natural sleep-wake cycle, resulting in insomnia or restless sleep. Beyond the physical realm, stress also affects our mental and emotional well-being. Anxiety and depression often accompany chronic stress, as the continuous activation of the stress response disrupts brain chemistry and mood regulation. Cognitive function may suffer, with memory lapses, difficulty concentrating, and impaired decision-making becoming more prevalent. Emotional regulation becomes challenging, leading to mood swings, irritability, and a sense of being overwhelmed by even minor stressors.

Managing stress effectively requires a multifaceted approach that addresses both the physiological and psychological aspects of the problem. Mindfulness practices, such as meditation and deep breathing exercises, offer tools for calming the mind and reducing the physiological arousal associated with stress. Regular exercise, healthy lifestyle habits, and social support systems all play crucial roles in building resilience and buffering against the negative effects of stress.

Furthermore, cognitive-behavioral techniques help reframe negative thought patterns and develop more adaptive coping strategies. Somatic movement practices, like yoga or tai chi, offer a holistic approach to stress management by releasing tension from the body and promoting relaxation.

In essence, Comprehending the Impact of Stress on the Human Body empowers us to take proactive steps towards managing it effectively. By adopting a comprehensive approach that addresses both the physical and emotional aspects of stress, we can cultivate resilience and maintain overall well-being in the face of life's inevitable challenges.

10.2 Stress-Reducing Breathing Techniques

Breathing is a powerful tool for managing stress and promoting relaxation. In this section, we'll explore several effective breathing techniques that you can easily incorporate into your daily routine to reduce stress and enhance overall well-being.

1. Diaphragmatic Breathing (Belly Breathing)

Description: Diaphragmatic breathing involves engaging the diaphragm muscle to take deep, slow breaths, filling the lungs completely with air.
Technique:
1. Lie down or find a comfortable sitting position.
2. Place one hand on your abdomen, just below your ribcage, and the other hand on your chest.

3. Inhale deeply through your nose, allowing your belly to rise as you fill your lungs with air. Feel your abdomen expand against your hand.
4. Feel your tummy drop as you slowly and fully exhale through your mouth, letting go of the breath in your lungs.
5. Continue this deep, slow breathing pattern for several minutes, focusing on the sensation of your breath moving in and out of your body.

Benefits: Diaphragmatic breathing activates the body's relaxation response, reducing stress hormones and promoting a sense of calmness and well-being.

2. Box Breathing (Square Breathing)

Description: Box breathing is a simple yet effective technique that involves breathing in a pattern of equal counts for inhalation, holding the breath, exhalation, and holding again, creating a "box" shape with the breath.

Technique:
1. Inhale deeply through your nose to a count of four, feeling your lungs fill with air.
2. For four counts, hold your breath while remaining relaxed and at ease.
3. Exhale slowly and completely through your mouth to a count of four, emptying your lungs of air.
4. Hold your breath again for a count of four before beginning the next inhalation.
5. Repeat this four-part breathing pattern for several cycles, focusing on the rhythmic flow of your breath.

Benefits: Box breathing helps regulate the autonomic nervous system, promoting relaxation, reducing anxiety, and improving focus and concentration.

3. Alternate Nostril Breathing (Nadi Shodhana)

Description: Nadi Shodhana is a yogic breathing technique that involves alternating the flow of breath between the left and right nostrils, balancing the body's energy and calming the mind.

Technique:
1. Sit comfortably with your spine tall and shoulders relaxed.
2. Tighten your right nostril with your right thumb.
3. Inhale deeply through your left nostril, counting to four.
4. Use your right ring finger to close your left nostril, and release your right nostril.
5. Exhale completely through your right nostril, counting to four.
6. As you count to four, take a deep breath through your right nostril.
7. Using your right thumb, shut your right nostril and open your left.
8. Exhale completely through your left nostril, counting to four.
9. Repeat this alternating breath pattern for several rounds, maintaining a steady rhythm.

Benefits: Nadi Shodhana promotes relaxation, clears the mind, and balances the flow of prana (life force energy) in the body.

4. 4-7-8 Breathing (Relaxing Breath)

Description: The 4-7-8 breathing technique, developed by Dr. Andrew Weil, is a simple practice that combines deep breathing and meditation, promoting relaxation and stress reduction.

Technique:
1. Begin by sitting or lying in a comfortable position, with your eyes closed.
2. Inhale deeply through your nose to a count of four, filling your lungs with air.
3. Hold your breath for a count of seven, allowing the oxygen to circulate throughout your body.
4. Exhale slowly and completely through your mouth to a count of eight, releasing any tension or stress with each breath.

5. Repeat this cycle for a total of four breaths, or as many times as needed to feel calm and relaxed.

Benefits: 4-7-8 breathing triggers the body's relaxation response, calming the nervous system, reducing anxiety, and promoting better sleep.

With practice, you'll develop the ability to harness the power of your breath to manage stress and enhance your overall quality of life.

10.3 Progressive Muscle Relaxation for Stress Relief

Progressive muscle relaxation (PMR) is a powerful technique for reducing stress and promoting relaxation by systematically tensing and then relaxing different muscle groups in the body. Let's explore this technique in detail and learn how to effectively practice it for stress relief.

Introduction to Progressive Muscle Relaxation

Progressive muscle relaxation was developed by Dr. Edmund Jacobson in the early 20th century as a method to help individuals reduce muscle tension and stress. The technique involves deliberately tensing specific muscle groups for a few seconds and then releasing the tension, leading to a deep sense of relaxation and calmness.

How Progressive Muscle Relaxation Works

PMR works on the principle of tensing and relaxing muscles to promote physical and mental relaxation. By deliberately tensing muscles and then releasing the tension, you can become more aware of the difference between tension and relaxation, allowing you to consciously release stress from the body.

Step-by-Step Guide to Progressive Muscle Relaxation

Follow these steps to practice progressive muscle relaxation:

1. Choose a Comfortable Position: Sit or lie down in a relaxed posture, keeping your legs straight and your arms at your sides. If you find it comfortable, close your eyes.

2. Deep Breathing: Breathe deeply for a few moments to help your body and mind relax. Breathe deeply through your nose to fill your lungs, then gently exhale through your mouth to let go of any tension or stress.

3. Tension and Release:

- **Start with Your Feet:** Concentrate on your toes and feet. Curl your toes down to tense the muscles in your feet. Hold the position for a little while, then let go of the tension entirely. As calm seeps through your feet, experience it.

- **Move to Your Calves and Thighs:** Gradually shift your focus to your calf muscles and thighs. Tense these muscles by pressing your heels into the ground and tightening your thigh muscles, then release the tension, allowing your legs to feel heavy and relaxed.

- **Continue Upward:** Progressively move upward through your body, tensing and releasing tension in each muscle group. Include your abdomen, chest, arms, shoulders, neck, and face. Tension should be applied to each muscle group for 5–10 seconds, followed by a 15–20 second release period.

4. Focus on Sensations: Observe your body's reactions as you contract and relax each muscle group. Allow yourself to completely release any residual stress or tension in your body as you become aware of the difference between tension and relaxation.

5. Repeat as Needed: Repeat the process of tensing and relaxing each muscle group as many times as needed to feel deeply relaxed and free of tension. With practice, you'll become more proficient at quickly achieving a state of relaxation.

Benefits of Progressive Muscle Relaxation

Progressive muscle relaxation offers numerous benefits for stress relief and overall well-being, including:

- **Reduced Muscle Tension:** By systematically tensing and relaxing muscles, PMR helps release built-up tension and stiffness in the body.

- **Stress Reduction:** PMR promotes relaxation of the mind and body, reducing stress hormones and promoting a sense of calmness and tranquility.
- **Improved Sleep:** Practicing PMR before bedtime can help you relax and unwind, leading to better sleep quality and more restful nights.
- **Enhanced Body Awareness:** PMR increases body awareness and mindfulness, helping you become more attuned to physical sensations and better able to manage stress.

As you practice regularly, you'll develop greater control over your body's response to stress and cultivate a deeper sense of peace and well-being in your life.

10.4 Mindfulness Meditation Practices for Stress Reduction

Mindfulness meditation is a powerful technique for reducing stress and promoting overall well-being by cultivating present-moment awareness and non-judgmental acceptance. Let's explore mindfulness meditation in detail and learn how to practice it effectively for stress reduction.

Introduction to Mindfulness Meditation

Mindfulness meditation is rooted in ancient Buddhist traditions but has gained widespread popularity in modern times as a secular practice for promoting mental and emotional health. It entails consciously focusing on the here and now without passing judgment, enabling you to examine your feelings, ideas, and physical experiences with acceptance and curiosity.

How Mindfulness Meditation Works

Mindfulness meditation works by training the mind to focus on the present moment, cultivating a state of heightened awareness and inner peace. By practicing mindfulness, you can learn to recognize and disengage from negative thought patterns and habitual reactions, leading to reduced stress and increased resilience.

Step-by-Step Guide to Mindfulness Meditation

Follow these steps to practice mindfulness meditation:

1. **Locate a Quiet Area:** Make sure the area you choose is peaceful, comfortable, and unoccupied. Sit or lie down in a relaxed position, with your spine straight and your hands resting comfortably in your lap or on your knees.

2. **Close Your Eyes or Soften Your Gaze:** Close your eyes if it feels comfortable, or simply soften your gaze and lower your eyelids to a half-open position. Allow your gaze to rest gently on a spot in front of you without focusing too intently.

3. **Focus on Your Breath:** As your breath enters and exits your body, pay attention to it. Observe how the breath feels entering and exiting your nostrils, as well as how your chest and abdomen rise and fall.

4. **Be Present:** Bring your attention to the here and now while you keep breathing. Without attempting to alter or interpret them, take note of any ideas, feelings, or experiences that come to mind. Just watch them with interest and an impartial awareness.

6. **Return to the Breath:** Whenever you notice your mind wandering or becoming distracted, gently redirect your attention back to your breath. When you need to refocus, use the breath as an anchor to help you return to the here and now.

7. **Practice Gratitude:** Take a few moments to cultivate a sense of gratitude for the present moment and for the opportunity to practice mindfulness. Acknowledge any feelings of contentment, peace, or joy that arise during your meditation.

8. **End with Compassion:** As you conclude your meditation, extend feelings of compassion and kindness to yourself and others. Wish yourself well and offer loving-kindness to all beings, recognizing our shared humanity and interconnectedness.

Benefits of Mindfulness Meditation

Mindfulness meditation offers numerous benefits for stress reduction and overall well-being, including:

- **Stress Reduction:** Stress can be decreased via mindfulness meditation, which encourages relaxation as well as a sense of composure and peace.
- **Improved Emotional Regulation:** By cultivating awareness of thoughts and emotions, mindfulness meditation enables you to respond to stressors with greater clarity and emotional resilience.
- **Enhanced Focus and Concentration:** Regular practice of mindfulness meditation can improve attention and concentration, leading to greater productivity and effectiveness in daily activities.
- **Increased Self-Awareness:** Mindfulness meditation enhances self-awareness and introspection, allowing you to gain insight into your thoughts, emotions, and behaviors.
- **Better Relationships:** By developing empathy and compassion through mindfulness meditation, you can improve your relationships with others and foster a greater sense of connection and understanding.

UNLOCK YOUR VITALITY:
SOMATIC MOVEMENT ROUTINES

11.1 Morning Somatic Routine

Start your day with this invigorating somatic routine designed to awaken your body and mind, setting a positive tone for the day ahead. Perform each exercise mindfully, focusing on your breath and sensations as you move through the sequence.

1. **Standing Cat-Cow Stretch (5 minutes):** Begin by standing with your feet hip-width apart. Inhale as you lift your arms overhead, arching your back gently and looking up towards the ceiling. Exhale as you bring your arms down, rounding your back and bringing your chin towards your chest. Repeat this flowing movement for 5 cycles, synchronizing your breath with your movements.

2. **Forward Fold with Ragdoll Arms (3 minutes):** From a standing position, exhale as you fold forward from your hips, keeping your knees slightly bent. Let your arms hang loosely towards the ground, allowing your head and neck to relax. Hold this position for 3 breaths, gently swaying from side to side if it feels good.

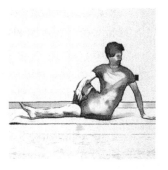

3. **Seated Spinal Twist (4 minutes):** With your legs out in front of you, take a seat on the floor. With your right foot on the outside of your left thigh, bend your right knee. Breathe in as you extend your back and out as you rotate to the right, extending your right arm behind you and resting your left elbow outside of your right knee. Hold the twist for 2 breaths, then repeat on the other side.

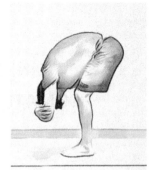

4. **Bridge Pose (5 minutes):** With your feet hip-width apart and your knees bent, lie on your back. Engage your thighs and glutes as you

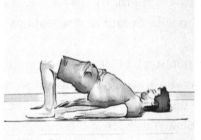

raise your hips toward the ceiling, pressing into your feet. For support, place your fingers below your lower back and bury your arms in the earth. After five breaths, leave the stance and gently lower yourself back down.

5. **Child's Pose (3 minutes):** Once you're kneeling on the floor, lean back on your heels and bend forward so that your arms are out in front of you and your forehead is resting on the floor. Take slow, deep breaths as you relax into the pose, allowing tension to melt away from your body.

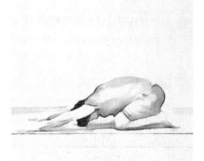

Take a break from your busy day to recharge and rejuvenate with this midday somatic routine. These simple exercises will help alleviate tension and boost your energy levels, leaving you feeling refreshed and focused for the rest of the day.

1. **Neck Rolls (2 minutes):** Sit or stand comfortably with your spine tall. Slowly lower your chin towards your chest and begin to roll your head in a clockwise motion, moving from ear to shoulder and then back around. After a few rotations, switch to counterclockwise. Repeat for 1 minute in each direction.

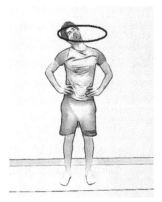

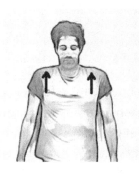

2. **Shoulder Shrugs (2 minutes):** Inhale as you lift your shoulders up towards your ears, then exhale as you release them down and back. Repeat this movement for 2 minutes, focusing on releasing tension from your shoulders and upper back.

3. **Side Body Stretch (3 minutes):** Stand with your feet hip-width apart and reach your arms overhead, clasping your hands together. Lean gently to one side, stretching through the opposite side of your body. Hold for a few breaths, then switch to the other side. Repeat this stretch for 3 cycles on each side.

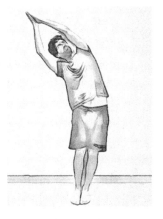

4. **Seated Forward Fold (4 minutes):** Sit on the floor with your legs extended in front of you. Inhale as you lengthen your spine, then exhale as you fold forward from your hips, reaching towards your feet. Keep your knees slightly bent if needed and hold the stretch for 4 breaths, feeling the lengthening of your hamstrings and lower back.

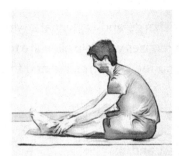

5. **Mindful Breathing (4 minutes):** Find a comfortable seated or lying position and close your eyes. Take slow, deep breaths, focusing on the sensation of the breath entering and leaving your body. Allow your breath to become smooth and steady, bringing a sense of calm and relaxation to your mind and body.

11.3 Evening Somatic Wind-Down

Wrap up your day with this calming somatic routine designed to promote relaxation and prepare your body for restful sleep. These gentle exercises will help release tension accumulated throughout the day, allowing you to unwind and let go of stress.

1. **Legs Up the Wall (5 minutes):** Lay flat on your back, making a 90-degree angle with your torso, and extend your legs up against a wall. With your palms facing up, place your arms by your sides. As you ease into the posture and feel the mild stretch in your hamstrings and lower back, close your eyes and take calm, deep breaths.

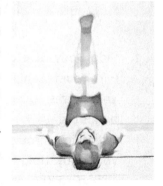

2. **Somatic Shoulder Release (3 minutes):** Sit or stand comfortably and reach your right arm across your chest, placing your left hand on your right elbow. Gently press your elbow towards your body,

feeling a stretch in your shoulder and upper back. Hold for a few breaths, then switch sides and repeat.

3. **Seated Twist (4 minutes):** Sit on the floor with your legs crossed or extended in front of you. Breathe in as you extend your back and out as you twist to the right, landing your right hand on the ground behind you and your left hand on your right knee. Hold the twist for a few breaths, then repeat on the other side.

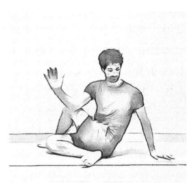

4. **Savasana (5 minutes):** With your arms and legs comfortably stretched and your palms facing up, lie on your back. Shut your eyes

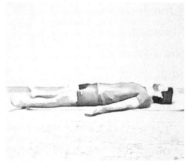

and let your body sink fully into the ground. Starting from your toes and working your way up to your head, concentrate on releasing tension from every muscle in your body. Remain in this pose for 5 minutes, breathing deeply and letting go of any remaining stress or tension.

5. **Mindful Body Scan (3 minutes):** Close your eyes and bring your awareness to your body. Begin at your feet and slowly scan upwards, noticing any areas of tension or discomfort. As you identify these areas, consciously relax and release them, allowing your body to sink deeper into relaxation with each breath.

Improve your flexibility and range of motion with this dynamic somatic mobility routine. These exercises focus on fluid movements to enhance joint mobility and overall physical function. Perform each movement mindfully, paying attention to the sensations in your body as you move through the sequence.

1. **Joint Circles (5 minutes):** Begin standing with your feet hip-width apart. Starting from your neck, gently circle each joint in your body, moving sequentially from your neck to your shoulders, elbows, wrists, hips, knees, and ankles. Perform 5 circles in each direction for each joint, focusing on smooth and controlled movements.

2. **Dynamic Forward Fold (4 minutes):** From a standing position, exhale as you hinge forward from your hips, reaching your hands towards the ground. Inhale as you rise back up to standing, sweeping your arms overhead. Repeat this movement for 4 cycles, coordinating your breath with the movement.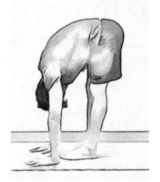

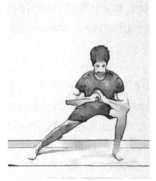 3. **Lateral Lunges (3 minutes):** Stand with your feet wider than hip-width apart. Shift your weight to one side as you bend your knee and lower into a lunge, keeping the opposite leg straight. Return to the center and repeat on the other side. Perform 6 lunges on each side, focusing on maintaining good alignment and stability.

4. **Spinal Waves (4 minutes):** Stand with your feet hip-width apart and soften your knees. Begin to articulate your spine, starting from your tailbone and moving sequentially through each vertebrae until your head drops forward. Reverse the movement, starting from your head and moving down towards your tailbone. Repeat this wave-like motion for 4 cycles, allowing your spine to move fluidly.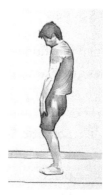

5. **Hip Circles (3 minutes):** Stand with your hands on your hips and your feet hip-width apart. Circle your hips in a clockwise direction, making smooth and controlled movements. After a few circles, switch to counterclockwise. Perform 6 circles in each direction, focusing on maintaining stability through your core.

6. **Figure 4 Stretch (4 minutes):** Sit on the floor with your knees bent 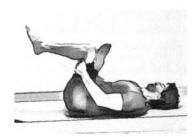 and feet flat on the ground. Cross your right ankle over your left knee, flexing your right foot. Lean forward slightly, feeling a stretch in your right hip and glute. Hold for a few breaths, then switch sides and repeat.

7. **Cat-Cow Stretch (3 minutes):** Place yourself on your hands and knees in a tabletop position. Take a breath and raise your tailbone and chest toward the ceiling by arching your back (cow position). Pull your chin in toward your chest and release the breath as you round your spine (cat stance). For six cycles, alternate between these two 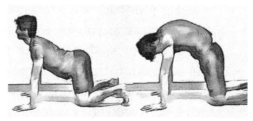 stances, matching your breath to your movements.

11.5 Somatic Strength Routine

Build functional strength and stability with this somatic strength routine designed to target major muscle groups while also improving coordination and body awareness. Perform each exercise mindfully, focusing on proper form and controlled movements.

1. **Somatic Squats (5 minutes):** Place your toes slightly out from your body and place your feet shoulder-width apart. Breathe in as you bring yourself down into a squat, maintaining your knees over your toes and your chest raised. Breathe out as you push through your heels to stand again. Focus on using your thighs and glutes as you complete 10 repetitions.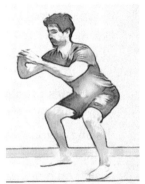

2. **Somatic Push-ups (4 minutes):** Begin in a plank position with your hands shoulder-width apart and core engaged. Breathe in while 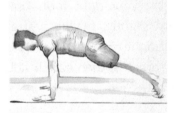 bringing your elbows close to your body and lowering your chest toward the floor. Exhale as you press back up to the starting position. Perform 8 reps, focusing on maintaining a strong and stable core throughout.

3. **Somatic Lunges (3 minutes):** Step your right foot back into a reverse lunge, lowering your back knee towards the ground. Inhale as you lower, then exhale as you press through your front heel to return to standing. Repeat on the other side. Perform 6 lunges on each side, focusing on proper alignment and stability.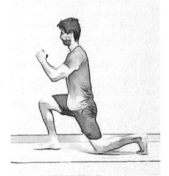

4. **Somatic Plank Variations (4 minutes):** Begin in a plank position on your hands or forearms, engaging your core and keeping your body in a straight line from head to heels. Hold the plank for 30 seconds, then transition to a side plank on your right forearm, stacking your feet and lifting your left arm towards the ceiling. Hold for 15 seconds, then switch to the other side. Repeat this sequence twice.

5. **Somatic Bridge (3 minutes):** With your feet hip-width apart and your knees bent, lie on your back. Taking a breath, contract your glutes and core, and raise your hips toward the ceiling. As you return to the beginning posture, release the breath. Perform 8 reps, focusing on maintaining a stable pelvis and avoiding arching your lower back.

6. **Somatic Side Leg Lifts (4 minutes):** Lie on your side with your legs stacked and your head supported by your bottom arm. Inhale as you lift your top leg towards the ceiling, keeping your hips stacked and core engaged. Exhale as you lower the leg back down. Perform 10 reps on each side, focusing on controlled movement and maintaining stability through your core.

Incorporate this somatic strength routine into your weekly workouts to build functional strength, improve stability, and enhance overall physical performance. Focus on proper form and controlled movements, gradually increasing the intensity as you progress.

11.6 Somatic Relaxation Routine

Promote deep relaxation and stress relief with this somatic relaxation routine designed to calm the nervous system and quiet the mind. Perform each exercise in a quiet and comfortable space, allowing yourself to fully relax and let go of tension.

1. **Somatic Breath Awareness (5 minutes):** Find a comfortable seated or lying position and close your eyes. Bring your awareness to your breath, noticing the rise and fall of your chest and belly with each

inhale and exhale. Breathe deeply and slowly, letting each breath out calm your body. Continue this mindful breathing for 5 minutes, focusing on the sensations in your body and the rhythm of your breath.

2. **Somatic Progressive Muscle Relaxation (7 minutes):** Begin by tensing the muscles in your feet, squeezing them tightly for a few seconds, then release and let go completely. Gradually work your way up through your body, tensing and releasing each muscle group, including your calves, thighs, glutes, abdomen, chest, arms, shoulders, neck, and face. Spend about 30 seconds on each muscle group, focusing on releasing tension and promoting relaxation.

3. **Somatic Body Scan (5 minutes):** Lie on your back with your arms and legs extended comfortably, palms facing up. Close your eyes and bring your awareness to your body. Starting from your toes, slowly scan upwards, noticing any areas of tension or discomfort. As you identify these areas, consciously relax and release them, allowing your body to sink deeper into relaxation with each breath.

4. **Somatic Mindfulness Meditation (8 minutes):** Find a comfortable seated position and close your eyes. Focus your attention on the here and now, observing any ideas, feelings, or sensations that surface without passing judgment. Allow yourself to simply be present, letting go of any worries or distractions. Focus on the sensation of your breath, using it as an anchor to keep you grounded in the present moment. Continue this mindfulness meditation for 8 minutes, allowing yourself to fully relax and unwind.

5. **Somatic Yoga Nidra (10 minutes):** Lie on your back in savasana, with your arms and legs extended comfortably, palms facing up.To fully settle into the posture, close your eyes and inhale deeply many times. Starting with your toes and working your way up to your head, start methodically relaxing every area of your body. As you

relax each body part, repeat a simple affirmation or sankalpa (intention) to yourself, such as "I am calm and at peace." Allow yourself to enter a state of deep relaxation and surrender, letting go of all tension and stress. Remain in this state of yoga nidra for 10 minutes, allowing your body and mind to experience complete relaxation and rejuvenation.

11.7 Somatic Cardio Routine

Elevate your heart rate and boost your cardiovascular health with this invigorating somatic cardio routine. These exercises focus on dynamic movements to increase blood flow, improve endurance, and enhance overall cardiovascular fitness. Perform each exercise with energy and enthusiasm, moving with intention and purpose.

1. **Somatic Jumping Jacks (5 minutes):** Start standing with your feet together and arms by your sides. As you simultaneously raise your arms high, jump with your feet wide apart. Lower your arms and jump back together to quickly return to the beginning position. Continue this jumping motion for 1 minute, focusing on landing softly and engaging your core muscles.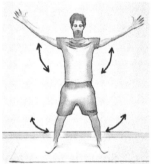

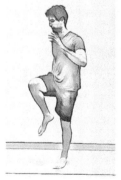 2. **Somatic High Knees (4 minutes):** Stand tall with your feet hip-width apart. Lift your right knee towards your chest as high as you can, then quickly switch legs, lifting your left knee towards your chest. Continue alternating legs as quickly as possible for 1 minute, pumping your arms to increase momentum and intensity.

3. **Somatic Butt Kicks (3 minutes):** Stand with your feet hip-width apart and arms by your sides. Flex your right knee and kick your right heel towards your glutes, then quickly switch legs, kicking your left heel towards your glutes. Continue alternating legs for 1 minute, moving at a brisk pace and focusing on bringing your heels towards your glutes with each kick.

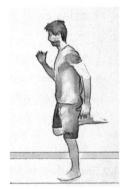

4. **Somatic Skaters (4 minutes):** Start standing with your feet together and knees slightly bent. Jump to the right, landing softly on your right foot with your left foot lifted behind you and your left arm reaching across your body towards your right foot. Quickly jump to the left, landing softly on your left foot with your right foot lifted behind you and your right arm reaching across your body towards your left foot.

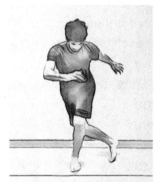

Continue jumping side to side for 1 minute, focusing on maintaining balance and agility.

5. **Somatic Mountain Climbers (3 minutes):** Start in a plank posture, with your body in a straight line from your head to your heels and your hands directly beneath your shoulders. Quickly alternate bringing your knees towards your chest, as if you are running in place while in a plank position. Continue this movement for 1 minute, keeping your core engaged and your hips stable.

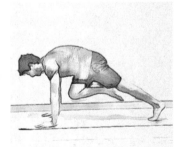

6. **Somatic Burpees (4 minutes):** Start standing with your feet hip-width apart. Squat down and place your hands on the ground in front of you, then jump your feet back into a plank position. Perform a push-up, then jump your feet back towards your hands and

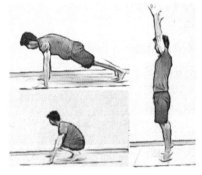

explosively jump up into the air, reaching your arms overhead. Land softly and immediately lower back down into the next rep. Perform as many burpees as possible for 1 minute, focusing on maintaining good form and intensity throughout.

11.8 Somatic Strength and Conditioning Routine

Build strength, power, and muscular endurance with this challenging somatic strength and conditioning routine. These exercises target major muscle groups while also improving stability, coordination, and functional movement patterns. Perform each exercise with proper form and control, focusing on quality over quantity.

1. **Somatic Squat Jumps (5 minutes):** Start standing with your feet shoulder-width apart. Lower yourself into a squat, then leap as high into the air as you can with great force. After a comfortable landing, quickly descend again to begin the next squat. Continue this jumping motion for 1 minute, focusing on generating power from your lower body and engaging your core muscles.

2. **Somatic Push-up Variations (4 minutes):** Start in a plank posture, with your body in a straight line from your head to your heels and your hands directly beneath your shoulders. Perform 10 regular push-ups, then transition into 10 tricep push-ups by keeping your elbows close to your body as you lower down. Finish with 10 wide

grip push-ups, with your hands positioned slightly wider than shoulder-width apart. Focus on maintaining proper form and control throughout each variation.

3. **Somatic Bulgarian Split Squats (3 minutes each leg):** Faced away from a sturdy elevated surface or bench, take a stand. With your left knee bent to around 90 degrees, take a lunge stance by placing the top of your right foot on the bench behind you. Push through your left heel to return to standing. Perform 10 reps on each leg, focusing on maintaining stability and balance throughout.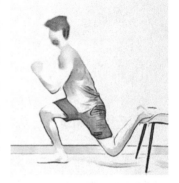

4. **Somatic Renegade Rows (4 minutes):** Start in a plank position on 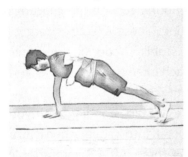 dumbbells or kettlebells, with your hands directly under your shoulders and your body in a straight line from head to heels. Engage your core and row the right weight up towards your right hip, keeping your elbow close to your body. Lower the weight back down and repeat on the left side. Perform 10 reps on each side, focusing on keeping your hips stable and avoiding rotation.

5. **Somatic Russian Twists (3 minutes):** Sit on the floor with your knees bent and feet flat on the ground. Using your sit bones for balance, slant your back a little and raise your feet off the ground. Hold a weight or medicine ball with both hands and rotate your torso to the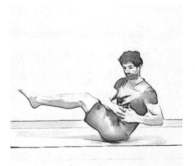

right, bringing the weight towards the ground beside your hip. Quickly twist to the left, bringing the weight towards the ground beside your left hip. Continue alternating sides for 1 minute, focusing on engaging your core and maintaining balance.

6. **Somatic Single Leg Deadlifts (4 minutes each leg):** Stand with your 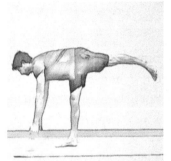 feet hip-width apart and knees slightly bent. Shift your weight onto your left foot and hinge at the hips to lower your torso towards the ground, extending your right leg behind you for balance. Keep your back flat and chest lifted as you lower down, then return to standing by squeezing your left glute and pressing through your left heel. Perform 10 reps on each leg, focusing on maintaining stability and control throughout.

11.9 Somatic Flexibility and Mobility Routine

Enhance flexibility, mobility, and range of motion with this comprehensive somatic flexibility and mobility routine. These exercises focus on gentle stretching and dynamic movement to improve joint health, reduce stiffness, and promote overall flexibility. Perform each exercise with ease and fluidity, moving mindfully and with intention.

1. **Somatic Dynamic Warm-up (5 minutes):** Start standing with your feet hip-width apart. Begin marching in place, lifting your knees towards your chest with each step. After 30 seconds, transition into arm circles, swinging your arms forward and backward in large circles. Continue alternating between marching and arm circles for 2 minutes, gradually increasing the range of motion with each movement.

2. **Somatic Cat-Cow Stretch (4 minutes):** Start on your hands and knees, placing your knees behind your hips and your wrists squarely beneath your shoulders. Take a breath, arch your back, raise your chest to the ceiling, and let your belly drop toward the floor 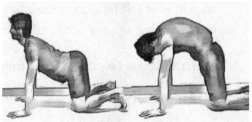 (cow posture). Breathe out as you draw your belly button toward your spine, tuck your chin into your chest, and curve your spine (cat stance). For two minutes, keep switching between the cat and cow poses, matching your breathing to your movements.

3. **Somatic Forward Fold (3 minutes):** Place your feet hip-width apart 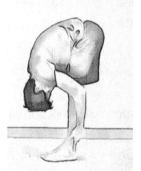 and stand tall. Breathe in while extending your arms aloft and lengthening your spine. Release the breath as you bend forward, extending your hands to your shins or the ground. If necessary, slightly bend your knees to keep your back flat. For one minute, hold the forward fold while concentrating on letting go of tension in your shoulders and neck and sensing the stretch in your lower back and hamstrings.

4. **Somatic Hip Flexor Stretch (3 minutes each side):** Kneel on your right knee with your left foot planted on the ground in front of you, creating a 90-degree angle with your left knee. Engage your core and gently press your hips forward until you feel a stretch in the front of your right hip. Hold the stretch for 1 minute, then switch sides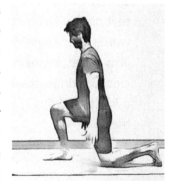

and repeat on the left side. Focus on maintaining a tall spine and avoiding overarching your lower back.

5. **Somatic Standing Quad Stretch (3 minutes each side):**Stand tall 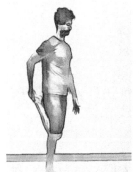 with your feet hip-width apart. Shift your weight onto your right foot and bend your left knee, bringing your left heel towards your glutes. Reach back with your left hand and grasp your left ankle, gently pulling it towards your glutes to deepen the stretch in your quadriceps. Hold the stretch for 1 minute, then switch sides and repeat on the right side. Focus on keeping your knees close together and your chest lifted throughout the stretch.

6. **Somatic Seated Forward Bend (4 minutes):** Sit on the floor with your legs extended in front of you and your feet flexed. Inhale as you lengthen through your spine, reaching your arms overhead. Exhale as you hinge at the hips and fold forward, reaching your hands towards your feet or shins. Allow your head to relax towards your knees and hold the stretch for 2 minutes, focusing on breathing deeply and relaxing into the pose.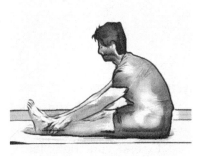

11.10 Somatic Senior Wellness Routine

Maintaining health and vitality is essential at every stage of life, especially as we age. This somatic senior wellness routine is designed specifically for older adults, focusing on gentle movements, balance exercises, and flexibility training to support overall well-being and quality of life. Perform each exercise with care and attention, listening to your body and honoring its limitations.

1. **Somatic Seated Marching (5 minutes):** Sit comfortably in a sturdy chair with your feet flat on the floor and your back supported. Lift your right knee towards your chest, then lower it back down and repeat with your left knee. Continue alternating between marching your knees for 1 minute, focusing on maintaining good posture and breathing deeply.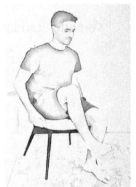

2. **Somatic Shoulder Rolls (3 minutes):** Sit tall in your chair with your 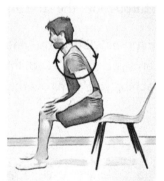 arms by your sides. Take a breath and raise your shoulders to your ears. Then, release the breath as you roll them down and back up in a gentle circle. Repeat for 1 minute, then reverse the direction of the shoulder rolls for an additional minute. Focus on releasing tension and promoting mobility in your shoulder joints.

3. **Somatic Leg Extensions (4 minutes):** Sit towards the front of your chair with your feet flat on the floor. Extend your right leg straight out in front of you, then flex your foot and hold for a few seconds before lowering it back down. For two minutes, alternate between the two legs and repeat with your left. Focus on engaging your thigh muscles and keeping your back supported throughout the movement.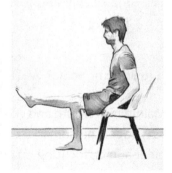

4. **Somatic Standing Balance (5 minutes):** Stand behind your chair and 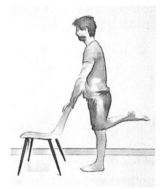 place both hands lightly on the backrest for support. Shift your weight onto your right foot and lift your left foot off the ground, balancing on your right leg for a few seconds. Lower your left foot back down and repeat on the other side. Continue alternating between legs for 2 minutes, focusing on finding stability and control with each balance.

5. **Somatic Chair Yoga Flow (8 minutes):** Sit back in your chair and take a few deep breaths to center yourself. Inhale as you reach your arms overhead, then exhale as you twist to the right, placing your left hand on the outside of your right knee and your right hand on the backrest of the chair. Hold the twist for a few breaths, then return to center and repeat on the other side. Continue flowing between seated twists, forward folds, and side stretches for 5 minutes, moving with ease and fluidity.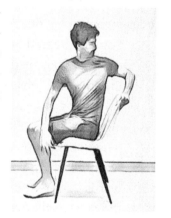

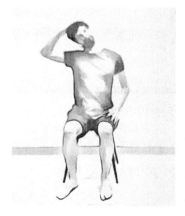

6. **Somatic Neck Stretches (3 minutes):** Sit tall in your chair and gently tilt your head to the right, bringing your right ear towards your right shoulder. Once you've held the stretch for a few breaths, go back to the middle and repeat on the left. Next, gently tilt your head forward, bringing your chin towards your chest to stretch the back of your neck. Hold

for a few breaths, then lift your head back up to center. Finally, tilt your head back slightly, opening up the front of your neck. Hold for a few breaths, then return to center. Repeat each stretch for 1 minute, focusing on releasing tension and improving mobility in your neck muscles.

11.11 Somatic Senior Gentle Stretching Routine

Maintaining flexibility and mobility is crucial for overall health and well-being, especially as we age. This somatic gentle stretching routine is designed to improve flexibility, reduce stiffness, and promote relaxation in older adults. Perform each stretch with slow, controlled movements, and focus on breathing deeply and mindfully.

1. **Somatic Seated Forward Fold (5 minutes):** With your legs out in front of you, take a comfortable seat on the floor or in a chair. Breathe in while extending your arms aloft and lengthening your spine. Exhale as you hinge at the hips and fold forward, reaching your hands towards your feet or shins. Hold the stretch for 2-3 minutes, allowing your head to relax towards your knees and your spine to lengthen with each breath. 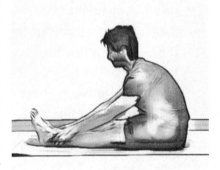 Focus on breathing deeply into your lower back and hamstrings, releasing tension with each exhale.

2. **Somatic Gentle Spinal Twist (4 minutes each side):** Sit tall in your chair or on the floor with your legs extended in front of you. Bend your right knee and cross it over your left leg, placing your right foot on the outside of your left knee. Inhale as you lengthen through your spine, then exhale as you twist to the right, placing

your left hand on your right knee and your right hand on the floor behind you for support. Hold the twist for 2 minutes, then switch sides and repeat on the left side. Focus on gently twisting from your waist, keeping your spine tall and your shoulders relaxed.

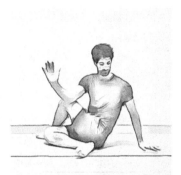

3. **Somatic Shoulder Stretch (3 minutes):** Sit or stand tall with your shoulders relaxed and your arms by your sides. Inhale as you reach your right arm overhead, then exhale as you bend your right elbow and place your right hand between your shoulder blades. Use your

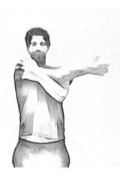

left hand to gently press your right elbow towards the midline of your body, feeling a stretch along the outside of your right arm and shoulder. Hold the stretch for 1-2 minutes, then switch sides and repeat on the left side. Focus on breathing deeply into the stretch, releasing tension with each exhale.

4. **Somatic Seated Side Stretch (3 minutes each side):** Sit tall in your chair with your feet flat on the floor and your arms by your sides. Inhale as you reach your right arm overhead, then exhale as you lean to the left, stretching your right side body. Hold the stretch for 1-2 minutes, feeling a gentle opening along the right side of your torso. Inhale to return to center, then repeat on the left side. Focus on elongating through your side body with each breath, finding length and space between your ribs.

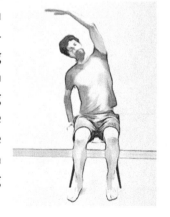

5. **Somatic Seated Hamstring Stretch (4 minutes):** Sit towards the front of your chair with your legs extended in front of you and your feet flexed. Breathe in as you stretch your spine; release the air as you bend forward at the hips and extend your hands to your shins or feet. Hold the stretch for 2-3 minutes, feeling a gentle stretch along the back of your legs. Focus on breathing deeply into your hamstrings, relaxing into the stretch with each exhale.

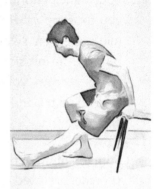

30-DAY SOMATIC TRANSFORMATION CHALLENGE: RELIEVE CHRONIC PAIN, SHED WEIGHT, AND ATTAIN MIND-BODY HARMONY IN LESS THAN 10 MINUTES A DAY

Welcome to the 30-Day Somatic Transformation Challenge! This challenge is carefully crafted to incorporate a series of targeted movements designed to increase body awareness and release accumulated muscle tension. These exercises focus on mind-body integration, encouraging the relaxation of chronic muscular tension through mindful movement. The primary goal of somatic exercises is to enhance posture, flexibility, mobility, and body awareness, thereby contributing to overall physical and mental well-being.

Day 1-5: Foundational Alignment

Day 1: Grounding Breathwork and Alignment

Today, focus on establishing a strong foundation through grounding breathwork and foundational alignment exercises. These practices center your mind and body, setting the stage for deeper somatic exploration.
Routine (10 minutes):
1. **Grounding Breathwork (2 minutes):** Sit comfortably, close your eyes, and take deep breaths to release tension.
2. **Neck Stretches (2 minutes):** To reduce tension in your neck, gently tilt your head from side to side.

3. **Shoulder Rolls (2 minutes):** Roll your shoulders to release tension in the upper back.
4. **Hip Circles (2 minutes):** Circle your hips to open and lubricate the hip joints.
5. **Spinal Twist (2 minutes):** Twist gently to each side to release tension in the spine.

Notice any changes in your body, breath, or state of mind. Establishing this foundation is vital for your somatic journey ahead. Enjoy the sense of presence and centeredness from mindful movement and breath.

Day 2: Gentle Neck Stretches

Today, we'll focus on releasing tension in the neck and shoulders through gentle, controlled stretches. These movements will help alleviate stiffness and promote relaxation in this commonly tense area.

Routine (10 minutes):

1. **Grounding Breathwork (2 minutes):** Start by sitting comfortably and taking several deep breaths to center yourself.
2. **Neck Flexion and Extension (2 minutes):** Slowly lower your chin towards your chest, feeling the stretch in the back of your neck. Then, gently tilt your head back, stretching the front of your neck.
3. **Neck Side Stretch (2 minutes):** To relax your neck, gently swivel your head from side to side.Raise your head to one side and press your ear to your shoulder until your neck's other side begins to gently extend.Repeat on the other side.
4. **Shoulder Rolls (2 minutes):** Roll your shoulders backward in a slow, controlled motion, focusing on releasing tension in the shoulder blades.
5. **Upper Back Stretch (2 minutes):** Interlace your fingers in front of you and round your upper back, stretching between the shoulder blades. Hold for a few breaths, then release.

Notice any sensations of release or relaxation in your neck and shoulders. Take a moment to appreciate the benefits of these gentle stretches and how they contribute to your overall well-being.

Day 3: Shoulder Rolls and Releases

Today, we'll focus on mobilizing the shoulders and upper back to promote relaxation and flexibility.

Routine (10 minutes):

1. **Grounding Breathwork (2 minutes):** Start by sitting comfortably and taking several deep breaths to center yourself.
2. **Shoulder Rolls (2 minutes):** Roll your shoulders backward in a slow, controlled motion, focusing on releasing tension in the shoulder blades.
3. **Shoulder Circles (2 minutes):** Extend your arms to the sides and make small circles with your shoulders, gradually increasing the range of motion. Reverse the direction after a minute.
4. **Upper Back Stretch (2 minutes):** Interlace your fingers in front of you and round your upper back, stretching between the shoulder blades. Hold for a few breaths, then release.
5. **Neck and Shoulder Release (2 minutes):** Sit or stand tall and gently tilt your head to one side, bringing your ear towards your shoulder. Place your hand on the opposite side of your head and apply gentle pressure to increase the stretch. Repeat on the other side.

Take a moment to notice any changes in the mobility and comfort of your shoulders and upper back. Appreciate the benefits of these movements in promoting relaxation and flexibility.

Day 4: Hip and Lower Back Mobility

Today, we'll focus on improving hip mobility and alleviating lower back discomfort with targeted exercises.

Routine (10 minutes):

1. **Grounding Breathwork (2 minutes):** Start by sitting comfortably and taking several deep breaths to center yourself.
2. **Hip Circles (2 minutes):** Stand with your feet hip-width apart and make slow circles with your hips, focusing on increasing the range of motion. Reverse the direction after a minute.

3. **Seated Spinal Twist (2 minutes):** Sit on the edge of a chair and place one hand on the opposite knee. Gently twist your torso towards the hand on the back of the chair, feeling a stretch in your lower back and hips. Hold for a few breaths, then switch sides.
4. **Forward Fold (2 minutes):** Position your feet hip-width apart, then bend forward at the hips to extend your reach toward your shins or the floor. Maintain a comfortable stretch in your hamstrings and lower back by bending your knees as much as necessary.
5. **Hip Flexor Stretch (2 minutes):** Step one foot back into a lunge position and lower your back knee towards the floor. Keep your front knee aligned with your ankle and gently press your hips forward to feel a stretch in the front of your hip. Hold for a few breaths, then switch sides.

Notice any improvements in the mobility and comfort of your hips and lower back after completing these exercises. Take a moment to appreciate the benefits of increased flexibility and reduced discomfort.

Day 5: Spine Alignment Practices

Today, we'll focus on aligning the spine and improving posture with gentle movements and stretches.

Routine (10 minutes):
1. **Grounding Breathwork (2 minutes):** Start by sitting comfortably and taking several deep breaths to center yourself.
2. **Cat-Cow Stretch (2 minutes):** Begin on your hands and knees, inhale as you arch your back and lift your head and tailbone towards the ceiling (cow pose). Inhale as you turn your back and adopt the cat stance, tucking your chin into your chest. Repeat for several breaths, moving fluidly between the two positions.
3. **Child's Pose (2 minutes):** From hands and knees, sit your hips back towards your heels and reach your arms forward, lowering your chest towards the floor. Relax and breathe deeply into the stretch along your spine.

4. **Standing Forward Fold (2 minutes):** Position your feet hip-width apart, then bend forward at the hips to extend your reach toward your shins or the floor. Lean your head back and let your spine extend.

5. **Seated Spinal Twist (2 minutes):** Stretch your legs out in front of you while you sit tall on the floor. Grasping the outside of your bent knee with your other hand, bend one knee and cross it over the other leg. Using your hand as support on the floor, twist your torso towards the bent knee. After holding for a few breaths, switch sides.

Take a moment to observe any changes in the alignment and comfort of your spine after completing these practices. Notice how these movements contribute to improved posture and overall well-being.

Day 6-10: Stress Relief and Emotional Balance

Day 6: Breathwork Integration

Today, we'll focus on combining breathwork with movement to enhance somatic awareness and reduce stress.

Routine (10 minutes):

1. **Grounding Breathwork (2 minutes):** To start, find a comfortable position and center yourself by inhaling deeply many times. Concentrate on taking deep breaths through your nose to fill your lungs, and then take slow, deep breaths out of your mouth to release any tension.

2. **Flowing Breath and Movement (4 minutes):** Stand with your feet hip-width apart. Breathe in as you extend your arms skyward, reaching for the stars. Breathe out as you fold forward, bending your knees if necessary, and lower your arms. Inhale to halfway lift, lengthening your spine, then exhale to fold deeper. Repeat this flowing movement for several breaths, allowing your breath to guide your motion.

3. **Seated Breath Awareness (2 minutes):** Sit comfortably with your eyes closed. Bring your attention to your breath, noticing the rise

and fall of your chest and abdomen with each inhale and exhale. Allow your breath to become slow and steady, anchoring you in the present moment.

4. **Mindful Walking (2 minutes):** Take a short walk, focusing on syncing your steps with your breath. Inhale as you take a step forward, and exhale as you bring the other foot to meet it. Pay attention to the sensations in your body as you move, staying present with each breath and step.

Take a moment to reflect on how combining breathwork with movement enhanced your somatic awareness and reduced stress. Notice any changes in your body and mind after completing this practice.

Day 7: Partner and Group Exercises

Today, we'll focus on connecting with others as we deepen our somatic practice through shared movements and support.

Routine (10 minutes):

1. **Partner Shoulder Stretch (3 minutes):** Pair up with a partner and sit back-to-back. Reach your arms behind you and clasp hands with your partner. Gently lean back, allowing your partner to guide the stretch in your shoulders and chest. Hold for a few breaths, then switch roles.

2. **Group Standing Twist (3 minutes):** Stand in a circle with your feet hip-width apart. Reach your arms out to the sides and twist your torso to the right, following the movement of the person next to you. Hold for a few breaths, then twist to the left. Repeat for several rounds, moving with the rhythm of your breath.

3. **Partner Forward Fold (4 minutes):** Sit facing your partner with your legs extended in front of you. Reach forward and clasp hands with your partner, then gently fold forward, allowing your partner to support you. After a few breaths, hold the stretch, then exchange positions.

Take a moment to reflect on how connecting with others through shared movements deepened your somatic practice. Notice any feelings of connection and support that arose during the exercises.

Day 8: Managing Stress and Anxiety

Today, we'll focus on learning somatic techniques to calm the nervous system and promote emotional well-being.

Routine (10 minutes):

1. **Grounding Breathwork (2 minutes):** Begin by sitting comfortably and taking several deep breaths to center yourself. Concentrate on taking deep breaths through your nose to fill your lungs, and then take slow, deep breaths out of your mouth to release any tension.

2. **Somatic Body Scan (3 minutes):** Close your eyes and bring your attention to your body. Start at your feet and slowly scan upward, noticing any areas of tension or discomfort. As you breathe, imagine sending relaxation and ease to each part of your body, allowing it to soften and release.

3. **Gentle Movement Sequence (3 minutes):** Stand with your feet hip-width apart and gently sway from side to side, allowing your arms to hang loosely at your sides. Feel the gentle rocking motion soothing your nervous system and promoting relaxation.

4. **Seated Meditation (2 minutes):** Find a comfortable seated position and close your eyes. Bring your attention to your breath, noticing the sensation of each inhale and exhale. As thoughts arise, simply acknowledge them and return your focus to your breath, cultivating a sense of calm and presence.

Reflect on how these somatic techniques helped to calm your nervous system and promote emotional well-being. Notice any shifts in your mood or state of mind after completing the practice.

Day 9: Emotional Release Practices

Today, we'll explore somatic practices for emotional release.

Routine (10 minutes):

1. **Body Scan Meditation (3 minutes):** Sit comfortably, close your eyes, and breathe deeply. Scan your body from head to toe, releasing tension with each breath.

2. **Shoulder and Neck Release (3 minutes):** Roll your shoulders and gently stretch your neck to release accumulated stress and tightness.

3. **Spinal Twists (2 minutes):** Sitting comfortably, gently twist your torso from side to side, allowing your breath to guide the movement and release tension in your spine.

4. **Child's Pose (2 minutes):** Sink into Child's Pose, stretching your arms forward and resting your forehead on the mat. Breathe deeply and allow any remaining tension to melt away.

Take a moment to notice any emotions or sensations that arise during the practice, and observe them without judgment or attachment.

Day 10: Cultivating Emotional Balance

Today, we'll focus on mindfulness and somatic awareness to cultivate emotional balance.

Routine (10 minutes):

1. **Mindful Breathing (3 minutes):** Find a comfortable seated position and close your eyes. Focus on your breath, inhaling deeply through your nose and exhaling slowly through your mouth.

2. **Body Awareness Scan (3 minutes):** Shift your attention to your body. Starting from your feet, gradually move your awareness upward, noticing any areas of tension or discomfort.

3. **Somatic Movement (3 minutes):** Begin moving your body in a way that feels natural and intuitive. Let your breath guide the movement, focusing on the sensations as you move.

4. **Seated Mindfulness (1 minute):** Return to a seated position, close your eyes, and bring your attention back to your breath. Take this moment to cultivate a sense of spacious awareness and presence.

After completing the practice, take a moment to reflect on any shifts in your emotional state or overall sense of well-being. Honor yourself for taking this time for self-care and reflection.

Day 11: Understanding Pain Relief

Today, we'll explore the connection between stress and physical discomfort, and learn techniques for relief.

Routine (10 minutes):

1. **Body Awareness Meditation (3 minutes):** Find a comfortable seated position and close your eyes. Bring your attention to any areas of tension or discomfort in your body, and breathe deeply into those areas, allowing them to soften and release.

2. **Neck and Shoulder Rolls (3 minutes):** Sit or stand tall, and gently roll your shoulders backward and forward. Then, tilt your head from side to side to release tension in your neck and shoulders.

3. **Breathwork for Pain Relief (3 minutes):** By taking a deep inhale via your nose, letting your belly expand, then gently exhaling through your mouth, you can practice diaphragmatic breathing. With each breath, visualize releasing any physical discomfort or tension.

Take a moment to reflect on how your body feels after completing the routine. Notice any changes in your level of discomfort or overall sense of well-being.

Day 12: Techniques for Alleviating Headaches

Today, we'll focus on addressing tension headaches and migraines with targeted somatic exercises.

Routine (10 minutes):

1. **Scalp Massage (3 minutes):** Using your fingertips, gently massage your scalp in circular motions, starting from the base of your skull and working your way up to your forehead. Focus on areas of tension and tightness.

2. **Neck Release Stretch (3 minutes):** Sit or stand tall, and gently tilt your head to one side, bringing your ear towards your shoulder. Hold for a few breaths, then switch sides. This stretch aids in the relief of upper back and neck strain.

3. **Shoulder and Upper Back Stretch (3 minutes):** Interlace your fingers behind your back and gently straighten your arms as you lift your chest and roll your shoulders back. Hold for a few breaths, then release. This stretch opens up the chest and relieves tension in the shoulders and upper back.

Notice any changes in the intensity or frequency of your headaches after completing the routine. Pay attention to how your body responds to the exercises, and adjust as needed.

Day 13: Managing Joint Discomfort

Today, we'll focus on easing joint pain and improving mobility through gentle, mindful movements.

Routine (10 minutes):

1. **Joint Circles (3 minutes):** Start by gently circling your wrists, ankles, knees, and hips in both directions. Focus on smooth, controlled movements and listen to your body's feedback.

2. **Cat-Cow Stretch (3 minutes):** Get on your hands and knees in a tabletop position. Breathe in as you raise your head and tailbone to the ceiling in the Cow Pose (arching your back); release the breath as you turn your spine and bring your chin up to your chest in the Cat Pose. Keeping the rhythm of your breath, repeat this action.

3. **Forward Fold with Knee Bend (4 minutes):** Stand with your feet hip-width apart and slowly fold forward from your hips, bending your knees as much as needed. Hold onto opposite elbows and let your head and arms hang heavy. Feel the stretch in your hamstrings, lower back, and shoulders.

Take a moment to notice any changes in your joint discomfort or range of motion after completing the routine. Notice how your body feels as you move through the exercises, and honor any sensations that arise.

Day 14: Incorporating Somatic Practices

Today, we'll focus on integrating somatic exercises into your daily activities for ongoing stress reduction and pain management.

Routine (10 minutes):
1. **Mindful Walking (3 minutes):** Take a short walk outdoors or around your home, focusing on each step and the sensation of your feet connecting with the ground. Pay attention to the movement of your body and any areas of tension or discomfort.
2. **Desk Stretches (3 minutes):** While seated at your desk, take a moment to stretch your arms overhead, interlace your fingers, and stretch side to side. Then, extend one leg at a time and flex your feet to stretch your calves and hamstrings.
3. **Somatic Breathing Break (4 minutes):** Sit comfortably and close your eyes. Take several deep breaths, focusing on expanding your belly with each inhale and fully exhaling any tension or stress with each exhale. Allow your breath to guide you back to a state of calm and relaxation.

Notice how incorporating somatic practices into your daily routine affects your overall sense of well-being and productivity. Pay attention to any changes in your physical and emotional state throughout the day.

Day 15: Workplace Wellness

Today, we'll explore strategies for promoting well-being and productivity in the workplace through somatic practices.

Routine (10 minutes):
1. **Seated Mindfulness Meditation (3 minutes):** Take a few moments to sit comfortably in your chair, close your eyes, and bring your attention to your breath. Notice the sensation of each inhale and exhale, allowing yourself to relax and center your mind.
2. **Desk Yoga (3 minutes):** Incorporate gentle yoga poses into your workspace by practicing seated twists, forward folds, and side stretches. Use your desk or chair for support as needed, and focus on releasing tension in your neck, shoulders, and back.
3. **Somatic Movement Break (4 minutes):** Stand up from your desk and take a short movement break. Shake out your arms and legs, roll your shoulders, and gently sway your body from side to side.

Allow yourself to move freely and release any built-up tension or stiffness.

Take note of how these brief somatic practices impact your focus, energy levels, and overall well-being throughout the workday. Consider incorporating them into your daily routine to support ongoing workplace wellness.

Day 16-20: Weight Loss and Physical Fitness

Day 16: Introduction to Weight Loss with Somatics

Today, we'll explore how somatic exercises can aid in weight loss and enhance body composition.

Routine (10 minutes):

1. **Body Awareness Meditation (3 minutes):** Begin by sitting comfortably and bringing awareness to your body. Notice any areas of tension or discomfort as you breathe deeply.

2. **Dynamic Standing Twist (3 minutes):** Stand with your feet hip-width apart and gently twist your torso from side to side, engaging your core muscles and promoting spinal mobility.

3. **Pelvic Tilt Exercise (2 minutes):** With your feet flat on the ground and your knees bent, lie on your back. Tilt your pelvis forward and backward gradually while contracting your abs.

4. **Body Scan and Visualization (2 minutes):** Close your eyes and scan your body from head to toe. Visualize yourself moving with ease and grace, embodying your ideal weight loss journey.

Take a moment to reflect on how somatic practices can support your weight loss goals and enhance your overall well-being.

Day 17: Warm-up Routine for Weight Loss

Welcome to Day 17! Today, we'll focus on preparing your body for exercise and optimizing calorie burn with a dynamic warm-up routine.

Routine (10 minutes):

1. **Neck Rolls (2 minutes):** Gently roll your neck in clockwise and counterclockwise circles, releasing tension in the neck and shoulders.
2. **Arm Circles (2 minutes):** With your arms out to the sides, adopt a tall stance. Using your arms, make little circles that progressively get bigger.
3. **Leg Swings (3 minutes):** Stand near a wall for support and swing one leg forward and backward in a controlled motion. Repeat on the other side.
4. **Torso Twists (3 minutes):** Stand with your feet hip-width apart and twist your torso from side to side, engaging your core muscles and warming up your spine.

Reflection: Notice how your body feels after completing the warm-up routine. Pay attention to any areas of increased flexibility or warmth.

Day 18: Core Strengthening Exercises

Today, we'll focus on engaging your core muscles to improve stability and support weight loss efforts.

Routine (10 minutes):

1. **Plank Hold (3 minutes):** Begin in a plank position, with your hands shoulder-width apart and your body forming a straight line from head to heels. Maintain good form and hold for as long as you can.
2. **Dead Bug Exercise (3 minutes):** Lay flat on your back with your legs bent 90 degrees and your arms reaching toward the ceiling. Slowly extend one leg outward while lowering the opposite arm behind you. Alternate sides.
3. **Bridge Pose (2 minutes):** Lie on your back with your knees bent and feet flat on the floor. Lift your hips toward the ceiling, engaging your glutes and core muscles. Hold for a few breaths, then lower down slowly.
4. **Russian Twists (2 minutes):** Sit on the floor with your knees bent and feet lifted off the ground. Hold a weight or medicine ball in

your hands and twist your torso from side to side, engaging your oblique muscles.

Take a moment to notice the activation of your core muscles during the exercises. Reflect on how these movements contribute to your overall strength and stability.

Day 19: Cool-down and Stretching

Today, we'll focus on promoting recovery and flexibility with a soothing cool-down routine.

Routine (10 minutes):

1. **Child's Pose (3 minutes):** Begin on your hands and knees, then sit back on your heels and extend your arms forward, resting your forehead on the mat. Breathe deeply and relax into the stretch.
2. **Seated Forward Fold (3 minutes):** Sit on the floor with your legs extended in front of you. Hinge at your hips and fold forward, reaching toward your feet. Hold the stretch and breathe deeply.
3. **Supine Spinal Twist (2 minutes):** Lie on your back with your knees bent and feet flat on the floor. T-pose with your arms out to the sides and your knees progressively lowered to one side while maintaining your grounded shoulders. Hold the stretch, then switch sides.
4. **Quad Stretch (2 minutes):** Lie on your stomach and bend one knee, bringing your heel toward your glutes. Reach back with one hand to grab your foot and gently pull it toward your body. Hold the stretch, then switch sides.

Notice how your body feels after completing the cool-down routine. Reflect on the importance of stretching for recovery and maintaining flexibility.

Day 20: Mindfulness Meditation Practices

Today, we'll focus on cultivating mindfulness to enhance self-awareness and mindful eating habits.

Routine (10 minutes):

1. **Seated Meditation (3 minutes):** Find a comfortable seated position and close your eyes. Focus on your breathing, taking slow, deep breaths through your nose and out through your mouth.
2. **Body Scan Meditation (3 minutes):** Shift your focus to your body, starting from your feet and gradually moving upward. Take note of any places where you feel tense or uncomfortable, then take a breath and let the tension and discomfort go.
3. **Mindful Eating Exercise (2 minutes):** Choose a small piece of food, such as a raisin or a piece of fruit. Take a few moments to observe it with all your senses before taking a bite. Notice the texture, taste, and sensations as you chew slowly and mindfully.
4. **Walking Meditation (2 minutes):** Step outside or find a quiet indoor space to walk slowly and mindfully. Pay attention to the sensation of your feet touching the ground with each step, and observe your surroundings with curiosity.

After completing the mindfulness meditation practices, take a moment to reflect on any shifts in your awareness or perception. Notice how these practices can support your journey toward mindful living and eating.

Day 21-25: Mind-Body Connection and Balance

Day 21: Understanding Stress and Its Effects

Today, let's deepen our understanding of stress and its effects on the body and mind.

Routine (10 minutes):

1. **Body Scan (3 minutes):** Begin by lying down comfortably. Close your eyes and bring your awareness to each part of your body, noticing any areas of tension or discomfort.
2. **Jumping Jacks (2 minutes):** Stand up and perform 1 minute of jumping jacks to get your blood flowing and release physical tension associated with stress.

3. **Breath Awareness (3 minutes):** Turn your attention to your breathing. Observe the innate cadence of your breaths in and out, without making an effort to regulate them.
4. **Gentle Movement (2 minutes):** Slowly transition into a seated position. Gently stretch your arms overhead and side bend from left to right, releasing any physical tension associated with stress.

Spend a moment reflecting on how stress manifests in your body and mind. Notice any insights or observations that arise from this practice.

Day 22: Stress-Reducing Breathing Techniques

Today, let's explore breathing techniques to reduce stress and promote relaxation.

Routine (10 minutes):
1. **Diaphragmatic Breathing (3 minutes):** Sit or lie down comfortably. Grasp your abdomen with one hand and your chest with the other. Breathe deeply through your nose, letting your stomach expand as air enters your lungs. As you slowly release the breath via your mouth, feel your belly drop.
2. **Alternate Nostril Breathing (2 minutes):** Sit comfortably with your spine tall. Take a deep breath through your left nostril and shut your right nostril with your thumb. Next, shut your left nostril with your right ring finger and release the breath via your right nostril. Continue this pattern for 1 minute, alternating nostrils with each breath.
3. **Squats (2 minutes):** Stand up and perform 1 minute of squats to release tension in your lower body and activate your leg muscles.
4. **Box Breathing (3 minutes):** Inhale deeply for a count of four, hold your breath for a count of four, exhale for a count of four, and then hold your breath out for a count of four. Repeat this cycle for 2 minutes, focusing on the rhythm of your breath.

Take a moment to reflect on how your body and mind feel after practicing these breathing techniques. Notice any shifts in your level of relaxation or mental clarity.

Day 23: Progressive Muscle Relaxation

Today, let's release tension and achieve deep relaxation through progressive muscle relaxation techniques.

Routine (10 minutes):

1. **Body Scan (2 minutes):** Begin by lying down comfortably. Close your eyes and bring your awareness to each part of your body, starting with your toes and gradually moving upward to your head.

2. **Progressive Muscle Relaxation (5 minutes):** Tense each muscle group in your body for 5-10 seconds, then release and relax completely. Start with your toes, then move to your feet, calves, thighs, buttocks, abdomen, chest, back, arms, hands, neck, and face.

3. **Forward Fold (3 minutes):** With your legs out in front of you, take a seat on the floor. Reach for your shins or toes as you slowly bend forward from the hips. Hold for 1 minute, breathing deeply into any areas of tightness or tension.

Notice how your body feels after practicing progressive muscle relaxation. Pay attention to any areas of lingering tension and observe the overall sense of relaxation in your body and mind.

Day 24: Mindfulness Meditation Practices

Today, let's deepen your meditation practice and cultivate present-moment awareness.

Routine (10 minutes):

1. **Seated Meditation (5 minutes):** Find a comfortable seated position, either on a chair or cushion. Close your eyes and bring your attention to your breath. Notice the sensation of each inhalation and exhalation, allowing thoughts to come and go without judgment.

2. **Body Scan (3 minutes):** Turn your focus to your body, examining it slowly from the top of your head to your toes. If you feel any tightness or discomfort, pay attention to those places and remove tension by breathing into them.

3. **Mountain Pose (2 minutes):** Stand tall with your feet hip-width apart and arms by your sides. Close your eyes and imagine yourself as a mountain, grounded and steady. Take deep breaths, feeling rooted to the earth with each inhale and reaching toward the sky with each exhale.

Take a moment to reflect on your meditation practice. Notice any changes in your ability to stay present and observe your thoughts without attachment. Acknowledge any distractions that arose during your practice and gently bring your focus back to the present moment.

Day 25: Mindfulness in Everyday Activities

Today, let's bring mindfulness into your daily life by practicing awareness in simple tasks and movements.

Routine (10 minutes):

1. **Mindful Walking (3 minutes):** Take a short walk outside or around your home, paying attention to each step you take. Take note of how your body moves with each step and how your feet feel on the ground.

2. **Mindful Eating (4 minutes):** Select a little snack, such a handful of almonds or a piece of fruit. Consider the food's flavors, textures, and colors for a moment before you eat. Chew carefully and enjoy the flavors as you take each bite, paying attention to the feelings in your tongue and body.

3. **Mindful Stretching (3 minutes):** Find a comfortable seated or standing position. Slowly stretch your arms overhead, lengthening through your spine. Take deep breaths as you stretch, feeling the expansion and release of tension in your body.

Reflect on how mindfulness enhances your experience of everyday activities. Notice any changes in your awareness, presence, and appreciation for the simple moments in life.

Day 26: Reflection and Gratitude

Today, we'll take a moment to reflect on our journey and express gratitude for our progress.

Routine (10 minutes):

1. **Neck Release Stretch (3 minutes):** Sit or stand tall and gently tilt your head to one side, bringing your ear towards your shoulder. Hold for a few seconds, then switch sides. Repeat 3 times on each side to release tension in the neck.
2. **Shoulder Roll Exercise (3 minutes):** Stand with your feet hip-width apart and roll your shoulders backward in a circular motion. After a few rotations, switch to forward shoulder rolls. Repeat for 3 minutes to release tension in the shoulders and upper back.
3. **Gratitude Journaling (4 minutes):** Grab a journal or a piece of paper and write down three things you're grateful for today. Reflect on how somatic practices have contributed to your well-being and growth.

Take a time to consider your trip thus far and recognize the strides you've achieved. Celebrate each step, no matter how small, and approach the remainder of the challenge with renewed gratitude and determination.

Day 27: Integration of Somatic Practices

Today, we'll focus on integrating somatic exercises into our daily routine for long-term health and well-being.

Routine (10 minutes):

1. **Seated Spinal Twist (4 minutes):** Place your legs out in front of you while sitting on the floor. Your right foot should be outside of your left knee as you bend your right knee. Place your left elbow outside of your right knee as you twist your torso to the right. After holding for a few breaths, switch sides. To increase spinal mobility, repeat for four minutes.
2. **Mindful Walking (6 minutes):** Take a mindful walk, paying attention to each step and the sensations in your body. Focus on the

connection between your feet and the ground, allowing your movements to be slow and deliberate. Walk for 6 minutes to integrate somatic principles into your daily routine.

Consider how you can continue to integrate somatic practices into your daily routine beyond the challenge. Explore ways to make movement and mindfulness a natural part of your lifestyle for sustained health and well-being.

Day 28: Self-Care Rituals

Today, we'll establish self-care rituals that nourish our body, mind, and soul.

Routine (10 minutes):

1. **Self-Massage (5 minutes):** Take time to give yourself a gentle massage, focusing on areas of tension or discomfort. Use slow, deliberate movements to promote relaxation and release.
2. **Deep Breathing Exercise (5 minutes):** Find a comfortable seated position and close your eyes. Take deep breaths, focusing on the sensation of air entering and leaving your body. Allow yourself to let go of any stress or tension with each exhale.

Reflect on the importance of self-care and how these simple rituals can contribute to your overall well-being. Commit to incorporating self-care practices into your daily routine moving forward.

Day 29: Celebration and Self-Compassion

Today, we'll celebrate our accomplishments and practice self-compassion as we continue our somatic journey.

Routine (10 minutes):

1. **Arm Circles (3 minutes):**Stretch your arms out to the sides while keeping your feet hip-width apart. Using your arms, create little circles that progressively get bigger. After a few rotations, switch directions. Repeat for 3 minutes to release tension in the shoulders and arms.
2. **Loving-Kindness Meditation (7 minutes):** Sit comfortably and close your eyes. Repeat phrases of loving-kindness to yourself,

such as "May I be happy, may I be healthy, may I be at peace." Extend these wishes to others as well, cultivating a sense of compassion and connection.

Take a moment to acknowledge your journey and all that you've accomplished. Offer yourself words of encouragement and kindness, knowing that each step forward is a testament to your strength and resilience.

Day 30: Somatic Transformation

Today, we'll embrace the transformative power of somatic practices and celebrate our newfound sense of vitality and balance.

Routine (10 minutes):

1. **Full-Body Stretch (5 minutes):** Dedicate this time to a full-body stretch, reaching your arms overhead and extending your legs long. Feel the energy flowing through your body as you release any remaining tension.

2. **Gratitude Practice (5 minutes):** Close your eyes and take a few deep breaths. Reflect on your somatic journey and express gratitude for the growth and transformation you've experienced. Visualize yourself moving forward with confidence and vitality.

Congratulations on completing the 30-Day Somatic Transformation Challenge! Take a moment to celebrate your achievements and acknowledge the positive changes you've made in your life. As you move forward, remember that the journey toward mind-body harmony is ongoing, and continue to nurture yourself with somatic practices and self-care.

CONCLUSION AND REFLECTIONS

In this final chapter, we reflect on the transformative journey you've embarked on through the world of somatic practices. We delve into the significance of your experiences, the lessons learned, and the path ahead as you continue to explore and integrate somatics into your life.

Acknowledging Your Progress

Take a moment to acknowledge the progress you've made since beginning this journey. Whether you're a beginner just starting out or someone who has been practicing for a while, each step forward is a testament to your dedication and commitment to your well-being.

Embracing Mind-Body Connection

Throughout this book, we've emphasized the importance of the mind-body connection in somatic practices. By tuning into your body's sensations, movements, and breath, you've cultivated a deeper awareness of yourself and how you move through the world. This connection forms the foundation for greater self-understanding and holistic wellness.

Celebrating Your Achievements

Honor your accomplishments, regardless of how minor they may appear. Whether it's mastering a new movement, experiencing relief from chronic pain, or simply finding moments of peace and relaxation, each success is a cause for celebration. By acknowledging and honoring your progress, you empower yourself to continue growing and evolving on your somatic journey.

Gratitude for the Practice

Express gratitude for the practice of somatics and the benefits it has brought into your life. From improved flexibility and mobility to enhanced emotional well-being and stress relief, somatic practices offer a wealth of benefits for both body and mind. Cultivating a sense of gratitude allows you to approach your practice with humility and appreciation for the transformative power it holds.

Looking Ahead

As you conclude this book, consider how you will continue to incorporate somatic practices into your daily life. Whether it's committing to a regular practice routine, exploring new techniques, or seeking out opportunities for growth and learning, the journey doesn't end here. Embrace the path ahead with curiosity, openness, and a willingness to explore the depths of your body and mind.

Final Words of Encouragement

In closing, remember that your somatic journey is unique to you. There may be challenges along the way, but with dedication, patience, and perseverance, you have the power to overcome them. Trust in your body's innate wisdom and continue to listen to its signals as you move forward. With each breath, each movement, and each moment of mindfulness, you are one step closer to embodying the full potential of somatic living. **Thank you for joining us on this journey of self-discovery and transformation. May your path be filled with peace, joy, and abundant well-being.**

Made in the USA
Las Vegas, NV
29 April 2024

89287969R00089